12 Steps t[illegible]ment Heaven

How to Plan for a Happy, Healthy and Meaningful Retirement

Second Edition

Table of Contents

First edition published - July 2022
Second edition published - April 2025

Preface to the Second Edition

It's been nearly three years now since I retired and I have been thinking for a while now about updating my book. So many things have changed in the political, social and economic landscape it was clear that many of the things in my original book were now out of date. Not to mention the fact that I have over three years of actual retirement experience now under my belt to speak of that I didn't have in the first book, which I suppose was more about researching and planning for retirement. I think my drive for the first book was born from my years of writing operating procedures in my role as manager of a hydro-electric scheme. It seemed right to have a guide book to refer to that would help myself and others who care to read it. In the second edition I attempt to simplify and provide longevity to some of the financial matters given that successive governments seem to continuously tweak and change things to suit their own political ends. Not great given that retirement can take decades of saving and planning for. I have also updated some of the non-financial sections based on feedback from readers, my own personal experience and further research and reading I have undertaken on the subject of retirement.

Prologue

'It's the journey, not the destination that matters' - T.S. Eliot.

It turns out there's actually 12 steps to heaven, despite the late Eddie Cochrane's 1960 song suggesting there were only 3. 12 steps to retirement heaven that is. Of course, whilst everyone's idea of retirement heaven will be different, what's more important is that you make sure to plan for it. Apparently many people spend more time planning their summer holiday than they do their retirement. You'll find lots of information and advice out there on the financial side of retirement planning but not so much on the personal and wellbeing side. This book is my personal journey into and exploration of retirement planning in the UK. Retirement can be a life changing experience, comparable to getting married, divorced, having a child, suffering a serious illness or injury or even being made redundant. So don't just let your retirement happen to you, make it happen for you and avoid ending up in retirement hell. Despite the title you don't have to be religious to get into retirement heaven. But you do need a plan. And you've made a good start by picking up this book to get you on track to a happy, healthy and meaningful retirement. So read on!

Are you wondering what retirement might look like for you? Are your reasons for retiring convincing you and your family? Are you worrying about how much money you will need, whether you have saved enough and what your pension options are? Have you thought about alternatives like semi-retirement, starting your own business or even doing some volunteering and what does that involve? What about setting a date for retirement? Is now a good time? Is what's happening with the global economic and political landscape likely to affect your decision? And what are you going to do with all of that extra time you'll have in retirement? Will you have fulfilling and meaningful things to do without a job to fill your day? And what about building a new routine outside of work? Are you worrying about how your physical and mental health and wellbeing will be affected by retirement? What about your social life, friends and relationships? How are you and your partner going to cope with all of that extra time you'll be spending together? Are your Wills and Powers of Attorney in order? And what about your retirement bucket list? Have you got one and if not what would you have on it? Well, if you're asking yourself these questions then you're on the right track, because these are all of the essentials that need to be considered and planned for when you are thinking about retirement. Or perhaps you've already retired and things haven't turned out quite as you had expected. But just because you can and want to retire, it doesn't necessarily always mean that you should. Especially if you're not properly prepared.

If I had a pound for every time someone asked me why I was retiring at 55 and what I was going to do with my time, I could probably have retired a year earlier. To be honest I hadn't really thought the answers through properly. Part of me also felt it was a little bit rude of people to ask me something I felt was quite personal. I often struggled with a reply and soon realised my answers were neither satisfying me nor my interrogators and I needed to put some more thought into it. So after a period of rumination I decided it would be a good idea to put my thoughts down on paper. And it ended up with me writing this book.

Of course everyone's answers to these types of questions will be different. For some it might just be because they can retire (financially speaking), for others it might be because they are bored and disillusioned with their job, or they want to try something new or start their own company and for others it might be due to redundancy or even for health reasons. The reality is it's probably a number of things coming together at the same time. When the stars align so to speak. Or when the scales are weighing more in favour of retirement than remaining in work. But as I said, just because you can retire, it doesn't always mean that you should! Have you thought about what else you are going to do? Whatever your reasons are, it's important you prepare well for your retirement. It's a major change in your life. So treat it with the due care and attention that it deserves.

Retirement used to happen when your employer or the state told you it was happening to you when you reached a certain age. Equality and Discrimination legislation now means you can now work for as long as you like or are able to work from a health perspective. Of course you still can't collect a state pension in the UK until you're of official retirement age, currently between 66 and 68 depending on when you were born but you can normally take a personal or company pension from 55, soon to be 57, again depending on when you were born. Whilst death in service benefits can be a generous employment perk for your family, it's probably not something you should be holding out for. Neither is holding out in the hope of a redundancy package in my opinion, unless it's imminent. I've seen too many people procrastinate on their retirement plans in the hope they would be made redundant. Being the author of your own destiny would be my best advice here.

The idea for the title of the book came from Jordan Peterson's 12 Rules for Life - An Antidote to Chaos. 12 is a good number to work with. There are 12 months in the year, 12 numbers on a clock face, 12 days of Christmas, 12 inches in a foot, Jesus had 12 disciples and King Arthur had 12 knights at his round table. Peterson talks about people having 7 basic 'needs' for a functional life:

1. friends and a family you get on with
2. an intimate relationship with someone you can trust
3. children
4. a job with prospects of promotion
5. a schedule
6. regulated use of intoxicating substances
7. having meaningful things to do in your spare time

Peterson says you need to be functioning well in at least 4 or 5 of these areas to be 'psychologically thriving'. However, retiring from work will mean losing 4 and initially 5 above so it's important you replace these and build on the others where possible.

I appreciate the discussions on pensions, living standards, care homes and legal matters are all complex and unique to the United Kingdom (also different in Scotland than the rest of the UK) and subject to change, however I have provided references in the Resources section at the end of the book to some of the topics discussed that you can refer to for updates on the current position. The majority of the remaining matters related to retirement planning, health and wellbeing, are I would say, universal. It's also important to state at the outset that I am not a qualified medical, legal or financial professional. The content of the book is based on my own personal experience, opinions, research and discussions I have had with other people who are already retired or who are looking to retire in the near future. It is important that you seek professional advice from a qualified medical practitioner, solicitor or independent financial advisor before making any changes, taking any actions or making any decisions that might have a detrimental impact on your health and well-being, legal or financial status.

But before we get into it, just remember you are retiring from work, not from life. Look forward to it like you would look forward to starting a new job, moving house, welcoming a new grandchild into the family or going on a big holiday. The end of one chapter in life and the beginning of another. Plan for it properly and you're in for a great retirement. Finally, and just to dispel the myth that early retirement can actually be bad for your health. A study from 2008 by Theo Nijman from the University of Tilburg concluded, ‘No negative effects of early retirement on men’s health’ (don't shoot the messenger ladies).

Step 1 - Why Should You Retire?

'He who has a Why to live can bear almost any How' - Freidrich Neitzsche.

An article in the Times from June 2022 by Ian King reported, 'the latest figures from the Office for National Statistics (ONS) suggested that overall economic inactivity rose by 522,000 people from October to December 2021 compared with the same months in 2019, immediately before the pandemic. Of those, about 493,000 were aged 50 or over. The ONS further reported that while some of them had given up work because of long-term illness or the need to look after family members, presumably in many cases suffering from Long Covid, the reason offered by most was **retirement**. Up to 221,000 people aged 50 or over gave this as their reason for leaving the labour force. This is particularly striking because it reversed a trend, established in the decade before the pandemic, in which a bigger proportion of workers aged 50 or over remained in the workforce for longer'.

My father died at the age of 48 when I was 18 and I have often looked back and thought it unfair that he died so young and lost the opportunities of seeing my brother and I grow into adults with successful careers, get married, have children of our own and generally live a long, happy and healthy life. Four years after my father died, my mother, at the age of 53, was diagnosed with a severe depression and anxiety disorder, a serious and debilitating life robbing condition she suffered with for the next 30 years. So your own personal life experiences will no doubt shape your answer to the 'Why' question. I've given some suggestions below to give you something to think about. Clearly the list is not exhaustive and some of these were my own reasons and some were reasons people have told me were theirs. You can decide on the ones that apply to you and no doubt you will have some to add of your own. Write down your own list and keep it handy for when you retire in case you have any thoughts of regret and need to refer back! But just because you think you have good reasons to retire it doesn't mean you should. There's still a lot more to think about.

Reasons for Retiring

- You've achieved financial independence - You've worked and saved hard all of your working life and you've accumulated the wealth you now deem sufficient to take you through your retirement years. Perhaps you can also supplement this income with some part time work. Perhaps you are able to cut back on your outgoings having paid off your mortgage, loans, etc and your children have flown the nest (be aware that departed hatchlings often come back as cash hungry adults). Perhaps you are also willing to sacrifice a little bit financially to pay for the freedom that retirement brings such as cutting down a little on your discretionary spending. Don't forget you're also likely to save on commuting costs. I cover financial matters in more depth in Steps 2 & 3 but achieving financial independence is a big factor if not 'the' biggest in anyone's reasons for retiring.
- You want to try something different - You're fed up with the same old routine and challenges your job is giving you. You're looking for new experiences, new challenges. You want to have time to pursue your own personal goals in life instead of being a slave to your employers goals. You want more time to spend doing things that benefit you and your family, not just your employers. You want to try some new hobbies or sporting interests. You might even want to move

house or move abroad or travel around the world in a campervan.

- You want to spend more time with family and friends - You probably spend more time with your colleagues than you do with your family. You're too exhausted at the end of the day to do anything other than watch TV. You want more time to engage and connect with family and friends in mutual hobbies and interests. You'd like to spend more time with your grandchildren. Maybe you could baby sit whilst their parents are at work. You have old friends you haven't seen in a long time and want to connect with them again.
- You're tired of commuting - You spend hours every day, stuck in traffic, having to deal with road rage and potholes or you're on unreliable, noisy, dirty public transport, listening to other passengers having annoying conversations on their mobile phones or engaging in other antisocial behaviour. Either way you're probably spending a fortune on fuel or public transport.
- You want to do some volunteering work - You want to put back something into society. Maybe you donate financially to charities and now you want to donate your time. Use the skills you possess to help others less fortunate. Raise funds for a favourite charity by doing some personal challenges.
- You want to retire whilst you're still in good health - You've given your employers the best and healthiest years of your life. You want to retain what is left of them for yourself. Or maybe you're suffering from poor health and you don't want to make things worse by continuing to work. You want to have additional time to improve your health by taking more exercise and engaging with new people outside of your work

circle. You want to spend more time outdoors, experience more of nature and improve your physical and mental health and wellbeing. You want to slow things down a bit. Get out of the fast lane and watch the world go by a bit. Let the younger ones carry the load.

- You have a poor work life balance - Can't relax and turn off from work, even on holiday. Constantly checking your phone for emails, WhatsApp and text messages during your time off work. Can't shrug off those guilty feelings of not being productive or efficient enough. Can't enjoy things during your time off, thinking about what's happening at work tomorrow or next week. Lacking attention span. Can't concentrate long enough to have a personal conversation, read a book, listen to music or watch a movie. Tired of multi-tasking.
- Your job has become too stressful, you feel undervalued or the type of work no longer suits you. You're burnt out. You're suffering from sleepless nights and tired of the endless emails, text messages, targets, stretch targets, ever reducing budgets, key performance indicators, deadlines, training courses, Teams calls, Zoom calls, Bored with doing the same thing every day. You've reached a career ceiling and further promotion is not worth the additional effort. You've accomplished all of your career goals. You're bored and have lost all motivation in your current role. You've got some difficult relationships with colleagues or overbearing, bullying or micromanaging bosses who think they can do your job better than you do. Your boss never gives you any feedback on your performance unless it's negative. No one covers for you when you're sick or on holiday

and you have a huge workload to come back to when you do.

- You're tired of woke company politics, ideologies and codes of ethics that don't fit with your own. You're rolling your eyes and biting your tongue at the corporate Environmental and Social Governance Policies, the Greenwashing, the corporate virtue signalling on Net Zero or Diversity, Inclusion and Equity (DIE) policies. The mandatory unconscious bias training. The Company takeovers, the restructures and the re-brandings. Most of which are done without your input, feedback or consent.
- Redundancy or ill health - Of course sometimes your retirement plans are taken out of your own hands. Redundancy might be a blessing in disguise if you are already close to retirement age or to reaching financial independence. If not then it might force you to seek out new employment for a period to tide you over. Redundancy is a difficult experience at any age but in the 50's plus bracket it can be difficult to re-engage with the employment market especially if you are going to be doing something different to what you are used to. The saying about teaching old dogs new tricks does have some validity in my experience, especially when it comes to learning new IT skills. Ill health or accidents of course can befall us at any time and again when you are older it can be harder to recover from these things. Sometimes life deals you cards you weren't expecting and you just have to play with the hand that you've been given.

Things You Will Miss About Work

You should also make a list of the things that you will miss about work. These are important as it will also provide you with some ideas for what to do in retirement. I cover this in more depth later in the book but it's worth jotting down a few ideas at this stage to make sure the seeds are planted, so to speak and you are beginning to think about plugging the gaps that retiring from your job will create in your life. Here are some suggestions about what you might miss about work to get you started:

- Financial Stability/Job Security - A salary payment that goes into your bank account every month, a bonus, a pension plan, paid holidays, healthcare, sick pay, sharesave schemes, a company car, cycle to work schemes. Are you ready for all of this to come to a sudden end on the day you retire? Have you made the necessary provisions to make sure you are comfortably financially independent, not only for now, but for the rest of yours and your partner's lives too?
- Friendship & Camaraderie - The relationships, friendships, trust, emotional support from work colleagues, built up over many years. Feeling part of a team, part of an organisation, part of a community. The opportunities to share personal stories with work colleagues, to socialise with them on nights out and then regret them on Monday mornings.
- Purpose, Meaning & Recognition - The satisfaction that comes with being good at your job or considered an expert in your own area. Being the person people come to for advice, instruction or mentoring. Receiving praise and thanks from a manager or colleague for a job well done. Taking on the challenges that work life brings. Being in a position of responsibility where you have a degree of influence over how the organisation is run, how its people are

treated and developed and how the business interacts with its shareholders, stakeholders, partners, customers, contractors, the media and the general public. How it manages its environmental and social responsibilities.

- Having a Sense of Identity - Having a job title you are proud of to tell people who ask you what you do for a living. Having a position of responsibility, not only in an organisation but also in society as a whole. Having a sense of worth, value and self esteem.
- Having a Routine - Knowing what you are going to be doing when you wake up each morning. Having a reason to get up and not just lie in bed all day. Having something to do each day without having to think too hard about it. Having things to fill your time that you might otherwise struggle with if you didn't have a job. Looking forward to the new challenges that each day at work will bring and also looking forward to coming home each evening. Looking forward to the end of the week and having the weekend off.

Retirement Alternatives

Or maybe after thinking everything through your reasons just aren't good enough yet, then you might want to consider some alternatives to retirement. So here are some suggestions for postponing or for easing yourself into retirement gradually:

- Reduce your hours - This is an excellent way of easing yourself into retirement as I discuss in Step 4. It lets you slow down a bit, frees up more time to help you develop more of your personal interests and reduces the responsibilities of a full time job.

- Change the things in your current job that are bothering you - Not an easy one but is it possible to negotiate a change to your job description to modify or remove the specific issues about your job that you don't like.

  (If your employer values you enough the above two options might be an alternative to them losing you completely).

- Change your Job - If your current employer won't let you reduce your hours and there are no options for altering your job description then you could always look for a different job with less working hours or less responsibility or working closer to home even. If you get an offer you could also use it as a negotiating tool with your current employer for a change of conditions.
- Start your own business/consultancy - Do you have skills, knowledge and experience you could sell to others. Do you want to be your own boss and work your own hours? Be aware that running your own business probably won't be an easy ride but if you're up for a challenge then what not. New IR35 rules have made life difficult for setting up as a sole trader or limited company so look into this if this is what you have in mind.

Whatever your thoughts are at this stage it's important you take plenty of time to think all of them through, weigh up the pros and cons about the various options described above including just staying where you are for the present and maybe reviewing everything again in a year's time. Make sure you discuss things with your family and take professional advice. It's a life changing decision so you need to make sure you consider all of the options and their implications and that your reasons are sound and robust for whatever decision you make. Because any decision that you do make could be irreversible. But in the end only you can decide what's best for you.

Step 2 - How Much Is Enough?

'Use money to gain control over your time, because not having control of your time is such a powerful and universal drag on happiness. The ability to do what you want, when you want, with who you want, for as long as you want to, pays the highest dividend that exists in finance' - Morgan Housel - Author of 'The Psychology of Money: Timeless lessons on wealth, greed, and happiness'. Morgan's book goes on to explain that financial success is less of a hard science but more of a soft skill, where how you behave (with money) is more important than what you know.

I often take delight in telling my own two children how well off they are now compared to how my brother and I were at their age. My mother worked as a shop assistant and a cleaner and my father had a number of relatively low paying self employed ventures. My earliest memories were of living in a one bedroom tenement flat in the east end of Glasgow with a single coal fire for heating and hot water, an outside toilet and only a small sink in the kitchen for washing in. We played in the streets, there were no clubs or organised activities. I had no idea how poor we were until I went to high school and made friends with children whose parents owned homes with gardens, fitted kitchens, bathrooms and separate bedrooms who also had cars and went abroad on family holidays. We didn't really go on family holidays together but I do remember going to my aunt's flat in London with my mother in the summer holidays. My uncle was the personal chauffeur to the Chairman of a large Chemical company whose HQ was based in London and they were lucky enough to have been given a flat to live in, as part of my uncle's job, that sat at the top of the company offices in Soho. These were great holidays and I have memories of my uncle picking us up from the train station in his boss's Rolls Royce. Also walking around London with my mother visiting all of the tourist attractions. We never had much money to spend other than the train fare down to London itself. My father never came with us but I do remember him ferrying me and his dogs around greyhound racing tracks all over Scotland in a tiny mini van in the 1970's that he had hand painted mat black. So whilst we were poor, I always remember us being happy, making the best of what we had, seeking out fun and adventure, not wasting anything, making things last and taking advantage of any opportunities that came our way. So how much is enough for you will probably depend on many factors, including your background, childhood and upbringing too.

It sounds like a no-brainer but probably the most important step in anyone's retirement plans is asking yourself if you can actually afford to. There's a rule of thumb that suggests you will need around 2/3 of what you were earning when you were working as an income in retirement. However, knowing exactly just how much you will need over the years that lie ahead isn't easy and everyone of us will have different commitments, spending habits, lifestyle choices, etc. so exactly 'how much' will be very dependent on the type of retirement you want to have. You will 'hopefully' have been saving hard for your retirement through pensions, savings, investments, property, etc and maybe you'll even have your own business. In retirement you will be moving from an asset accumulation phase to an asset drawdown phase. Or eating the nuts you've been squirrelling away for the past decades. The important question to ask yourself is have you squirrelled away enough nuts to endure the years that lie ahead?

Another rough rule of thumb of working out how much you will need as a pension in retirement is to calculate your annual expenses and multiply it by 20. So if you need £25,000 per annum then your pension should be roughly £500,000. This equates to a drawdown rate of 4% over 30 years of retirement. I talk about the 4% drawdown rule further on.

Obviously when your monthly salary stops getting paid into your bank account, this income source will need replacing with pensions or savings to cover your ongoing expenses. At first this might seem a frightening prospect. I know it was for me. Especially when you look at your gross salary. I kept asking myself, is this something I'm prepared to give up. I was earning a decent salary and had other perks like a car allowance, private health care, sick pay and an annual bonus. Of course when I deducted tax and national insurance it was significantly less! So it's the net salary figure you want to focus on. Of course when you do retire your income tax is likely to reduce, you'll no longer need to pay National Insurance contributions and you'll no longer be paying into a pension. You are also likely to have paid off or be close to paying off your mortgage, your children might have completed their education or even be working. In addition you won't have work commuting costs so overall your ongoing expenses and commitments will be reduced. Don't worry if you don't tick all of these boxes though. The main thing is that you account for them in your financial planning calculations. If you do still have a mortgage or outstanding loans to pay off you will want to consider if you want to keep paying these through your retirement income or if you just want to pay them off using savings or using your pension tax free lump sum. Starting with a clean sheet sounds better to me.

You can also make additional savings in retirement if you are willing to drop your living standards a notch. Doing some of your own DIY, booking 3* rather than a 4* hotels (my wife strongly disagrees with this one), going on one foreign holiday a year instead of two, going out for lunch rather than dinner (avoiding the alcohol bill), shopping at Aldi and Lidl instead of Waitrose and M&S, cutting down to one car or downsizing your existing car, downsizing your house and using the additional time you will have to seek out the bargains and other ways of saving money.

I suppose you need to decide on the type of retirement and lifestyle you want to live. Are you prepared to sacrifice your living standards a little to gain the additional time and freedom that retirement brings? When you are working you are effectively exchanging your freedom (or time) for money. You can continue to exchange your time for money for as long as you are fit to work however you can't do it the other way around. You can't buy back time in retirement. Your time on this earth is limited and finite. But only you can decide when the scales tip in favour of more time and freedom instead of more money.

Needs, Wants and Aspirations

So the next thing to work out is what your expenses are going to be in retirement. Start with your short term non-discretionary living expenses like food, gas, electricity, transport, council tax, rent, insurance policies, education fees, property maintenance, etc. You can call these your financial **Needs**. The non-discretionary things that you can't avoid paying for basically. You can use your bank and credit card statements over the last 12 months as a starting point for calculating these.

Next up is to determine your financial **Wants**. Consider these as your short term annual discretionary expenses like holidays, entertainment, home improvements, etc. Add your Needs and Wants together and this will be your total annual budget requirement.

And finally you can also think about longer term expenses such as replacing cars, supporting children/grandchildren through private school or higher education or helping them with car or house purchases, weddings, buying a camper van and travelling around the UK or Europe, taking cruises, buying a holiday home, building a home extension or even moving abroad. Call these your **Aspirations**. You can also refer to the bucket list ideas in Step 12 for this one. Whilst care home fees might not be aspirational, they should be considered as part of your long term expense plans too.

The Pensions and Lifetime Savings Association PLSA provides minimum, standard and comfortable living standards for singles and couples in the UK. The budget areas (basket of goods) considered included food, alcohol, tobacco, clothing, water rates, council tax, insurance, fuel, other housing costs, household goods, household services, personal goods and services, motoring, other travel costs and social and cultural participation. Table 1 summarises the findings. Bear in mind these numbers are after tax so the actual figures required will be higher when grossed up. So where do you fit in this table with your own standard of living? Do these budgets meet your needs and can you afford it?

Table 1 - Retirement Living Standards in UK in 2024

Retirement Living Standard	**Single Person Annual Budget**	**Couple Annual Budget**
Minimum	£14,400	£22,400
Moderate	£31,300	£43,100
Comfortable	£43,100	£59,000

Source - www.retirementlivingstandards.org.uk

Work Out Your Net Wealth

It's also drawing up an asset balance sheet of your total accumulated wealth including pensions, savings, investments, your home, rental properties, businesses, personal property, jewellery, cars, together with any debts, loans and other liabilities. It's useful knowing your net wealth as it's likely not just to be your pension you'll have as an asset to live off in retirement and you may want to crystallise different assets as different stages of your retirement so as to minimise income tax, capital gains tax, inheritance tax and to maximise investment gains. So how much is the average Household and Individual Net wealth in the UK? Well, according to nimblefins.co.uk, in 2022, Table 2 shows what it looks like for age groups 50+.

Table 2 - Household & Individual (Net) Wealth in the UK by Age Group in 2022

Average Household Wealth by Age	**Age 50-54**	**Age 55-59**	**Age 60-64**	**Age 65+**
Financial Wealth - Cash, Savings, ISA's	£59,700	£81,700	£116,900	£113,600
Pension Wealth	£309,000	£417,900	£483,700	£275,600
Property Wealth	£208,000	£250,000	£283,000	£284,000
Physical Wealth, personal items, jewellery, art, cars, etc	£58,300	£60,700	£63,500	£57,300
Total Average Household Wealth	**£635,100**	**£810,000**	**£947,600**	**£730,900**
Individual Wealth	**£305,337**	**£405,000**	**£473,550**	**£309,824**

Source - nimblefins.co.uk

So, once you've worked out your net worth and how much you're going to need in retirement, then it's time to have a look at your pension options.

Die with Zero

Die with Zero, a book by Bill Perkins on 'Getting All You Can from Your Money and Your Life' is a personal finance book with a unique philosophy that encourages readers to prioritize experiences and memories over hoarding wealth. The book challenges conventional approaches to saving and spending, advocating for a life of intentional living and maximizing fulfillment. Here's a summary of the key ideas:

Core Principles:

1. **Maximize Life Experiences:** Perkins argues that money is best spent on experiences that bring joy and create lasting memories. He urges readers to allocate resources to experiences during the prime years of life when they can be fully enjoyed.
2. **Focus on Time and Health:** The book emphasizes that time and health are more finite than money. Perkins encourages people to evaluate their spending decisions based on their current ability to enjoy life, as waiting too long could mean missing out.
3. **Die with Zero:** The central concept is that the goal should be to spend down one's wealth during their lifetime to avoid leaving behind unused resources. Perkins suggests planning finances so that wealth is consumed at the optimal time for maximum happiness.
4. **The Power of Memory Dividends:** Perkins introduces the idea of "memory dividends" — the long-lasting joy and value we derive from past experiences. Investing in memorable experiences pays dividends for years in the form of happiness and satisfaction.
5. **Avoid Over-Saving:** Many people save excessively for retirement, fearing they'll outlive their money. Perkins provides strategies for balancing saving with spending, using tools like annuities to ensure financial security without sacrificing enjoyment.

6. **Bucket Your Life:** Perkins suggests dividing life into stages or "time buckets" and planning experiences for each stage based on age, health, and ability.
7. **Optimize Giving:** Rather than leaving an inheritance, Perkins advocates for giving to loved ones or charities while alive. This allows you to witness the impact of your generosity.
8. **Take Risks While You Can:** The book encourages taking calculated risks earlier in life when there's more time to recover from setbacks. This approach can lead to greater opportunities and richer experiences.

Practical Advice:

- **Track Your Life Experiences:** Make a list of things you want to do and allocate resources to achieve them.
- **Decumulate Wealth:** Plan for a gradual reduction of wealth over time, ensuring you have enough for your needs but not excessive surplus.
- **Reassess Life Regularly:** Continuously adjust your plans to align with changing priorities, health, and circumstances.

Philosophy: At its heart, *Die with Zero* is about living intentionally, avoiding regrets, and ensuring that wealth serves as a tool to enhance life rather than an end goal. Perkins invites readers to redefine success, focusing on living a rich and meaningful life rather than merely accumulating financial security.

Step 3 - What are Your Pension Options?

'There's no pensions for old prize fighters' - Jake LaMotta.

How Much 'Can' You Save Into Pension

In April 2019 the minimum contributions to auto-enrolment workplace pensions were raised to 8% of earnings, including 3% employer and 5% employee contributions. But even this is unlikely to give you the pension pot you will need for a comfortable retirement. You only receive tax relief on personal contributions. Employers' contributions do not receive tax relief.

The amount of tax relief you get depends on what you earn each year:

- Earnings of £3,600 or less - you can put in up to £2,880 into a pension each year and it will be topped up with up to £720 in tax relief.
- Earning between £3,601 and £12,570 - you can put 100% of your earnings into a pension each year (including employee & employer contributions and tax relief).
- Earning £260,000 or less - you can put up to 100% of your earnings or £60,000, whichever is lower, into your pension (including employee & employer contributions and tax relief).
- Earning over £260,000 - your annual limit lowers by £1 for every £2 of income that goes over £260,000. So, if you're earning £300,000, for example, you will only only get tax relief on the first £4,000 you put in your pension each year.

Be aware of the Money Purchase Annual Allowance (MPAA) rules which will reduce the maximum amount you can contribute into a pension from £60,000 to £10,000 if you decide to take any taxable income from your pension. This does apply to taking tax free cash only.

You can also carry over any unused contribution allowance from the previous three tax years and pay it into a pension assuming you have the earnings in that year to cover it.

How Much 'Should' You Save into a Pension

www.finder.com reported 'the average pension savings in the UK stand at just £35,357 per person in 2023, including both retired and non-retired adults. This is down from an average pension pot of £42,651 in 2021, a decrease of 17%. To enjoy a moderate standard of living on retirement at age 66 in 2023, it is recommended to have £285,000 saved in total. However, the average UK adult has only 12.4% of this saved in their pension pot. How many people have a pension? Less than two-thirds of adults (58%) stated that they had pension savings in our survey. Almost 1 in 5 adults (18.4%) either do not have a pension of any kind or have nothing saved into their pension, which is estimated to be 9.7 million people. A further 16% of people are unsure how much they have saved in their pension. What is the average UK pension pot at retirement? According to survey results, retired people have £69,481 saved in their pension pot on average. This is approximately a quarter (24.4%) of the recommended UK retirement income for a moderate standard of living of £285,000'.

Source: https://www.finder.com/uk/pensions/pension-statistics

Analysis conducted by finder.com

Martin Lewis of moneysavingexpert.com also has a 'very rough' rule of thumb which suggests that the amount of money you should be saving into your pension as a percentage of your gross salary should be 50% of your age when you start saving to put you into a strong pension position. So if you start saving at 25 years old then you should be saving 12.5% of your gross salary into your pension.

For a more sophisticated approach there are plenty of retirement savings calculators available online. The one I have used for the example below can be found at www.moneyhelper.org.uk

Retirement Savings Example

A single male aged 25 and earning the 2024 average UK salary of £35,828 per year, looking to retire on 2/3 of his salary (inclusive of the state pension and before tax is taken off) and assuming he retires at the age of 68 would need to save 11.2% of his gross salary assuming he also receive the 3% minimum employer pension contribution. This assumes pension contributions will increase in line with inflation and pay rises at 2.5% each year, they will receive tax relief, investments will grow by 5% each year, charges will be 0.75% each year and he will have made full National Insurance contributions for at least 35 years. The pensions calculator tool at moneyhelper.org.uk is very useful and allows you to use slider bars to adjust personal & employer contributions, retirement age, target income in retirement and salary to help you determine your own personal sweet spot for pension planning.

State Pension & Pension Reforms

In 1765 the average life expectancy (combined for men and women) in the United Kingdom was below 39 years. In 2020, two and a half centuries later, it had increased by more than double, to 80.9 (79.0 years for men and 82.9 years for women). When the Old Age Pension was introduced in 1909, for people aged 70 and over, the average life expectancy was about 51. If you were lucky enough to still be alive at 70, your state pension would have been around 5 shillings per week (around £27 in today's money) or 7 shillings and sixpence a week for a couple (£40 in today's money) and the pensions were subject to a means test. It wasn't until 1946 and through the National Insurance Act that a State Pension for everybody was implemented on a contributory basis. Taking effect from 1948, men were eligible at 65, whilst women could receive it at 60. In 2010 the State Pension age started to change for women, beginning its increase from 60 to eventually 65 in line with men.

Currently the state pension age in the UK is 66 for both men and women however two further increases have been set out in legislation – a rise to 67 for those born on or after April 1960 should come into effect by 2028 and a rise to 68 for those born on or after April 1977. The full rate of the new State Pension at Oct 2024 is £221.20 per week or £11,502 per year for those reaching State Pension age on or after 6 April 2016. The state pension increases each year in line with the highest of average earnings, prices - as measured by inflation - and 2.5 percent. This is known as the triple lock. You will usually need at least 10 qualifying years on your National Insurance record to get any State Pension and 35 qualifying years to get the full State Pension and you will get a proportion of it if you have between 10 and 35 qualifying years. One of the major gripes of this system is that once you have paid the 35 years of national insurance contributions (NIC's) you need to get a full state pension, you don't stop paying NIC's if you continue working and no further benefits are accrued to your state pension. So if you live to the average age in the UK of 80.9 (male and female combined) you can expect to receive 14.9 years of state pension, assuming you've paid NIC's for 35 years. You can check what state pension you are entitled to using the HMRC website at www.gov.uk/check-state-pension

Many people say the UK state pensions are poor due to a measure used by the Organisation for Economic Co-operation and Development (OECD) known as the replacement rate, which shows how much of your earned income is replaced by the state pension when you retire. In the UK this is 58% (the OECD average is 62%) This means that on average about 58% of our retirement income comes from the state and 42% from workplace pensions, savings etc. In 2023/24 the UK spent about 5..1% of its GDP on state pensions, pension credit and winter fuel payments.

The Financial Services Act came into force in 1988 and personal pension plans were also launched in the same year. In 2015 further pension reforms were introduced, including the age at which a private pension could be accessed increased from 55 to 57 from 2028 and would then remain at 10 years below the State Pension age. From the age of 55, you can access as much of your savings from your defined contributions pension scheme (also known as 'money purchase schemes') as you want to, under new 'pensions flexibility' rules.

Defined Contribution & Self Invested Personal Pensions

Defined Contribution (DC) and Self Invested Personal Pensions (SIPP's) (also commonly referred to as workplace stakeholder and personal pensions) where the amount you get when you retire depends on how much you and/or your employer put into them, tax relief, where it is invested and how much the investments grow. Under current UK rules, employees earning at least £10,000 must be auto-enrolled into a company's pension scheme if they are aged between 22 and the state pension age. By law their employer then has to make contributions of at least 3% of their salary with the employee adding 5%. Pension funds are normally invested in the stock market amongst other investments so their value can fluctuate. If you have a DC or SIPP type pension, one option when you retire is to purchase an Annuity. This is a policy that allows you to swap a lump sum for a guaranteed income in retirement. This is what most DC/SIPP pension savers had to do before pension rules were relaxed in 2015. You had to buy an annuity with some or all of your pension pot. Annuities are insurance products that offer a set payout for life in exchange for a lump sum, so you can buy yourself a guaranteed income in retirement. How much you will be offered will depend on interest rates at the time, your age, your health and the type of annuity you choose, however only 10% of retiring investors bought an annuity in 2020-21, according to the UK City regulator, the Financial Conduct Authority. In 2023/24 however there was a 39% increase from the previous year due to a rise in annuity rates, which made them more attractive to retirees.

Alternatively you can use what is called a pension drawdown facility. This allows you to take a lump sum from your pension fund of up to 25% tax fee and then draw down an annual income on the remaining balance. A rough rule of thumb (discussed in the 4% Rule below) is that every £100,000 saved in a DC or personal pension can provide you with £4000 of annual pension income assuming a 4% drawdown rate. The 4% figure is discussed as being a limit to ensure your pension pot does not run out during a 30 year retirement period but this depends on inflation and investment growth too so your drawdown rate should be regularly reviewed. The benefits of a drawdown pension is your drawdown rate can be flexible to suit your needs at the time. You might need more in the earlier years to support dependents and a more active lifestyle and less in later years or when you start to receive the state pension. So for example you could draw down 4.5%, 4% and then 3.5% reducing by 0.5% every 10 years over a 30 year retirement period. There are plenty of online pension drawdown calculators where you input the size of your pension pot, your attitude to investment risk, estimated growth rate, inflation rate and it will tell you how long your pension might last. I have included one from Which in the Resources section.

Defined Benefit (DB) - Final Salary Pension

These schemes were commonplace in the second half of the 20th century (and are still used largely in the public sector and some ex-public sector companies), but declined significantly at the start of the 21st century in the private sector as the costs associated with these schemes increased substantially. These cost increases were driven by various factors, including an increase in life expectancy, the dot-com bubble burst, a reduction in bond yields and increasing regulation. Instead of building up a pension pot over time like a DC pension, a DB pension can provide you guaranteed annual income for life (like an annuity), usually based on either your final salary or career average salary, the number of years you have worked with the company (hence the name) and a multiplication ratio, normally 1/60 or 1/80. So for example if you retired on earnings of £50,000/year, having worked for 40 years and your pension had a 1/60 ratio, you might expect to get an annual pension of 40/60 x £50,000 = £33,333. In a DB scheme you are also allowed to take a tax free lump sum up to 25% and a smaller pension on the remaining balance instead. This can be useful if you are keen to avoid the higher rate tax brackets. With a DB pension scheme you will normally get the guarantee of an inflation linked pension income until you die, after which your spouse might get a reduced pension (usually 50% of what you were receiving) until they die. However with a DB pension, similar to an annuity but unlike a DC pension, there is no residual inheritance value to the pension to pass onto your children.

The 4% Rule

The 4% rule is a simple rule of thumb to help you avoid running out of money in retirement. It says that you can withdraw 4% of your savings in your initial year of retirement and adjust that amount for inflation for each subsequent year without the risk of running out of money for about 30 years. It might sound good in theory and it might work for some in practice but if you're blindly following this formula without considering whether it's right for your situation, you could end up either running out of money or being left with a financial surplus that you could have spent on other things. The 4% rule assumes your investment portfolio has a 60/40 percent stock/bond ratio split and assumes you'll maintain your spending level throughout retirement at 4% of your savings. If this is true for you and you want to follow a simple retirement withdrawal strategy, then the 4% rule might work for you.

But if you want to be sure you won't run out of money, following the 4% rule might not be the best option. It doesn't really account for changing markets. In a period of economic recession, high inflation or stock market downturns for example you might want to reduce withdrawals and when things improve in the economy, you might be able to withdraw more than 4%. Also, if you've not chosen an asset mix of 60/40 stock/bonds then you should avoid following the 4% rule, because this is the asset mix that the rule was based on. When you invest differently, your portfolio will perform differently. For example, investing more in bonds could result in slower investment growth because bonds typically don't see the returns that stocks do. If you're expecting your spending patterns to change throughout retirement, the 4% might not be the best approach either. You are likely to be more financially active in the early part of your retirement with hobbies, travelling, supporting dependents, etc, with spending then falling in mid-retirement, and then rising later in life with healthcare costs. So the 4% might not be flexible enough to account for the different retirement phases and limits you to a set amount, which might not be enough in your early years and might be too much in your later ones.

Transferring DB Pensions

An alternative introduced in 2015 pension reforms allowed DB pensions to be transferred into Self Invested Personal Pensions SIPPs to allow greater flexibility on how you could access your pension. This meant trading off the benefits of an index linked pension for life with one that would be subject to the performance of the stock market. One of the benefits of transferring out of a DB scheme is that it becomes an asset that can be passed on (currently free) of inheritance tax to the family. It also offers the flexibility of taking a higher income in the early years when it is more needed which can then be reduced in the later years. There has been negative publicity of DB pension transfers due to the scandal at British Steel where about 8000 employees collectively transferred about £2.8bn from the firm's scheme when it was restructured in 2017. The Financial Conduct Authority states that, for most consumers it's not in their best interests to transfer out of a Defined Benefit pension. Where a consumer seeks advice to transfer, firms must give suitable advice that is personalised to their needs and situation. If advice is unsuitable, consumers can suffer harm. Some may end up with less money in retirement, with no guarantee about the amount of income available at retirement. If you are considering transferring a DB pension and it is valued at over £30,000, then by law you will be required to take financial advice. I've included a link in the Resources section to further information on DB pension transfers.

Tax Free Allowances in Retirement

Okay the good news is you don't pay National Insurance on your pension withdrawals. You will however still have to pay income tax on your pension withdrawals (excluding your 25% tax free element) however there are ways to minimise this. You could use up any personal savings or ISA's to begin with first before drawing down your pension. You can also draw down up to £16,750 per year from your pension and not pay any tax at all using your 25% tax free allowance. So you can take £4,190 from your 25% tax free allowance and the balance of £12,570 as drawdown income which will be tax free under your annual personal allowance.

Be aware that taking all of your tax free lump sum in one go, unless you really need if to pay off your mortgage for example, is that once you have taken your money out of the pension tax free wrapper then depending on where you invest it, any interest, dividends or capital gains received on your lump sum will likely be taxable. The maximum tax free amount you can withdraw from your pension will be 25% of the 'now abolished' lifetime allowance of £1,073,100, (so £268,275).

The UK Government also changed inheritance tax rules in Oct 20024 meaning that pensions will now be considered as part of your estate for inheritance tax purposes from April 2027 although you can still transfer pensions, inheritance tax free, between spouses/civil partners.

But remember your other tax free allowances:

- £500 dividends allowance
- £1000 personal savings allowance
- £5,000 starter rate savings allowance
- £3000 capital gains tax allowance
- £1,000 trading allowance
- £1,000 property allowance
- £7,500 rent a room allowance
- £20,000 ISA allowance
- £50,000 Premium Bonds allowance

Investment, Diversification and Market Volatility

Having a diversified portfolio means spreading your risk geographically, across different industries and across different asset classes such as bonds, shares, properties, currencies and commodities. Essentially this means not having all of your eggs in one basket but instead having a range of investments which are not all equally affected by the same things at the same time. Remember you are already invested in property if you own your own home or a rental property. Depending on your attitude to risk, a balanced portfolio could have 60 per cent in a globally diversified mix of private company shares and 40 per cent in mixed global bonds. A 60/40 global index tracker fund might tick all the boxes for a diversified portfolio however it all depends on your appetite for risk.

Negative stock market returns do occur, but historical data shows that the positive years outweigh the negative years. In any given year, the actual return you earn may be quite different from the long-term average return, which averages out several years worth of performance. One indicator of market conditions is the Buffet (Warren) Indicator, which is a ratio of the value of all publicly traded US securities as a percentage of American GDP. When the indicator is high it means stocks are expensive. It stood at 160% in June 2022 which is around twice the level at which Buffet suggests that stocks might be a bargain. One way to lower your exposure to market volatility is to drip-feed your money into investments over time. This pound-cost averaging means that you buy consistently, regardless of whether the prices are low or high.

The other important thing to remember about being invested in the stock market, as your pensions are likely to be, is that you remain invested for the long term. Try not to focus too much on the daily fluctuations of the markets or trying to time the market by selling high and buying low or even worse selling investments when they are falling and thereby crystallising your losses. History has shown that good investment management is about the length of time in the market rather than trying to time the market.

Pensions Advice

Pension Wise is a government service from moneyhelper.org.uk that offers free, impartial pensions guidance about your pension options. An appointment with Pension Wise is free and will help you understand what your overall financial situation will be when you retire. It'll talk you through your options to help you make the right decision. You can also seek independent financial advice. There might be aspects of your lifestyle that you have not yet considered, which may influence your investment strategy. An IFA is trained to probe into your finances as a whole, and so recommend the best approach or even recommend that investing is not the best route for you personally. You don't have to agree, but their unbiased opinion is worth having and the first appointment is normally free. An IFA can also help you to choose the best asset classes and recommend the best funds available for your needs. Unless you want to, you won't have to invest from scratch, picking individual stocks – your IFA can select suitable products from the whole of the market. Your IFA can also manage the investment admin side of things.

Managing your Own Pension

If you'd rather go it alone, Pete Mathew's meaningfulacademy.com website runs online training courses for people at various points in their financial life stages. In his retirement planning course he talks about setting up a cash flow ladder within your pension in retirement where he suggests setting up separate investment buckets for the different stages of your retirement depending on your attitude to risk and your financial needs. The idea being you have separate investment buckets for the years ahead of you with the level of investment risk increasing as the years progress on the basis that your riskier investments will have time to recover should they suffer a stock market crash and you won't be selling assets that have dropped in value for immediate cash needs. So for example, if your annual pension need was say £30000, then your years 1-2 bucket should hold £60000 in cash, on the basis that cash will be unaffected by any stock market fluctuations. Cash of course will still be subject to inflation and interest rates however this will be significantly less volatile than stock market investments. With years 3-5 bucket you could take a little bit of a risk with say holding £90,000 in a 20/80 or 40/60 (bond/equity) multi asset global tracker fund, perhaps having separate investments for bonds and equities. With years 6-10 bucket you could take a little more risk with say £150,000 in a 60/40 or 80/20 tracker fund and beyond year 10 you might want to go with 100% equities. There is a one off fee for taking the Retirement Planning Academy but this also gives you access to the 'Voyant Go' retirement planning tool, for an ongoing fee, which is a very useful and powerful program to help you with your long term financial planning. Pete Mathew also provides free YouTube videos and a Podcast which are both very helpful and recommended.

In Summary

There is a lot of information and advice out there to be found on the financial aspects of retirement both free and paid for. The main takeaway from this step is to make sure you work out what your expenses are going to be, short and long term, work out the net value of your assets, review the various options available to you for accessing pensions and crystallising your assets to provide you with a retirement income in a way that minimises your tax burden and maximises how long your funds will last whilst at the same time making sure you don't leave too mech that will be taken as inheritance tax when you die. Bearing in mind your expenses at the start of your retirement are likely to be higher and needed for different things than they will be in the middle before perhaps rising again at the end of your retirement. There are also longer term financial planning matters to consider such as capital gains tax, inheritance tax and care home fees potentially. Obviously you will have more time to think about and plan for these matters but it's important to give some thoughts to them as well the important Wills and Power of Attorney documents and I cover this in Step 11. And finally please do consider independent financial advice before taking any actions or decisions that once they are made may become irrevocable.

Step 4 - When Should You Retire?

‘Progress only starts when you get clear on where you are right now’ - Michael Hyatt

For most people the biggest factor influencing the ‘when’ question will be dictated mainly by the affordability question. But again, just because you can afford to retire, doesn't always necessarily mean you should!

At the time of writing, the average retirement age in the UK was 64.55 years with women retiring on average 1.1 years earlier than men. A significant number of workers living in London can expect to be working into their 70s and 1 in 10 workers in the East Midlands usually give up work before they hit 60. In France it's 62, in Germany and Finland it's 65, in the United States it’s 62, in Mexico it's 69, in Japan it’s 70 and in South Korea it’s 72. Meanwhile members of the FIRE Movement (Financial Independence Retire Early) have aspirations of retiring in their 40’s!

According to the ONS, about half a million people aged 50 and over left work between 2019 and 2021 after more than 10 years of high investment returns. But they were not to know what impact a global pandemic followed by a global energy crisis and the Russian invasion of Ukraine would have had on the economy or their finances. 39% per cent now say they would consider returning to work and 52% cite money as their main reason.

Getting older brings thoughts of your own mortality and how long you think you might have left. The WHO defines healthy life expectancy (HLE) as the ‘average number of years that a person can expect to live in "full health" by taking into account years lived in less than full health due to disease and/or injury'. According to the ONS, in the UK in 2017 to 2019, HLE at birth in the UK for males was 62.9 years, showing no significant change since 2014 to 2016; however, HLE for females showed a significant decrease from 63.7 years in 2014 to 2016 to 63.3 years in 2017 to 2019. **Full** life expectancy (FLE) at birth in the UK in 2018 to 2020 was 79.0 years for males and 82.9 years for females; this represents a fall of 7.0 weeks for males and almost no change for females (a slight increase of 0.5 weeks) from the latest non-overlapping period of 2015 to 2017. In Scotland in 2018-2020, full life expectancy at birth was 76.8 years for males and 81 years for females. Working to the current state pension age of 67 would leave a man on average 9.8 years of life expectancy. The current average HLE age for a man from Glasgow (my hometown) is only 54. Glaswegians also have a 30% higher risk of dying before they are 65 (considered a premature death) than people in comparable de-industrialised cities such as Liverpool and Manchester. They die from the big killers: cancer, heart disease and strokes, as well as the "despair diseases" of drugs, alcohol and suicide. You can also consider how old your parents and grandparents and their siblings are and how healthy they were in their later years. So full life and healthy life expectancy are important considerations. I have provided a link to the ONS website in the Resources section which provides you with an online personal life expectancy calculator if you provide your age and sex. I've never liked to miss an opportunity but my family missing out on cashing in on my company's 'Death in Service' insurance policy hasn't been a big disappointment to me. Retiring in a good state of physical and mental health makes sense. You don't want to let your job completely run you into the ground. Do you?

Are you planning on retiring at the same time as your spouse/partner? Is it a good idea for you both to make such big changes at the same time? Are you going to be happy spending a lot more time together? Don't underestimate the rates of 'grey' divorce in the 50's plus group (more on this in Step 9). Can you afford to both retire at the same time? Personally I chose to take a reduction to my working week in my final year at work and split the extra time off I had between the days my wife was at home and the days she would be working, so it was a good system for us and allowed us to gradually adjust to seeing more of each other around the house during the day and building a new routine together. My wife is 5 years younger than me and so at the time I chose to retire at 55, my wife was still 5 years away from the minimum retirement age so retirement wasn't really on her mind. That didn't mean it wasn't an easy task convincing her that it was a good idea that I should retire early whilst she continued working for another 5 years! And do prepare to take on additional household chores when you are at home and your partner is working. Obviously!

Redundancy is another potential opportunity to take early retirement. It might come unexpectedly and earlier than you'd planned for but redundancy might just help tip the scales, financially speaking, as to whether you can afford to retire earlier than planned. The electricity supply industry has seen its fair share of this over the last two decades with the closure of many coal and nuclear power stations in the UK and for many of the people I knew it came at the right time and helped provide an early retirement for them.

You might even want to align your retirement with a milestone in your life. Some people on final salary pensions may decide to retire at the point where they have maximised their qualifying years. So if their final salary pension was based on a 40/60 of their final salary they might leave after 40 years service with the company as this was the maximum period they could benefit from from their final salary pension. Other milestones could be the minimum age for withdrawing a pension of 55 or your 60'th birthday or even the state retirement age.

The 'When' question isn't an easy one and you could make the case there's never a good time to retire. There are so many things outside your sphere of influence that if you are waiting for all of the stars to align in your favour it will be your funeral, not your retirement, you're planning for. Here's a list of some notable global events of the last 20 years that might have made you think twice about retirement had you know about them in advance:

2001 - Terrorist attacks on the WTC in New York and the subsequent invasion of Afghanistan and hunt for Ossama Bin Laden
2003 - Invasion and war in Iraq in the hunt for WMDs and removal of Saddam Hussein
2005 - London terrorist bombings and 80,000 killed in an earthquake in Kashmir
2008 - Stock market crash and start of a global recession
2009 - H1N1 Swine flu pandemic kills an estimated 284,000
2010 - Earthquake in Haiti in 2010 kills 230,000
2011 - The world's population reached 7 billion
2016 - UK votes to leave the EU and America votes for Donald Trump as president
2017 - A terrorist attack at an Ariana Grande concert in Manchester kills 22 and injures over 140
2020 - Covid 19 global pandemic and stock market crash with a death toll of 5.95 million in Feb 2022
2021 - World Leaders declare a Climate Emergency at the COP Summit in Glasgow and the US withdraw troops from Afghanistan causing global unrest and further human mass migration into Europe

2022 - Russia invades Ukraine. Energy prices & inflation rates soar across the world

All of the above of course are completely out of your control and predictability. So whilst these types of events might make you worry about the future, there's not really anything you can do personally about them except to decide in the moment if this is the right time to retire or to hold out a little bit longer, make better preparations and see how things pan out.

There are also of course lots of personal and family reasons you could cite to defer retirement - children leaving school or university, getting their first jobs or getting on the housing ladder, (repeat all of this with grandchildren too), looking after elderly parents. No doubt you can add to this list.

Finally you should also consider when is the best time of year to retire. Retiring in mid winter when the weather is cold and wet and there's not much daylight probably isn't a great idea. Especially if you're planning on spending more time outdoors on hobbies. Probably best to plan to finish up during the spring and summer months and not end up stuck indoors for the first six months of your retirement, but then again it comes down to personal preferences here. So when is the right time to retire exactly? Well only you can answer that question.

Step 5 - Slowing Things Down

'Taking time to do nothing often brings everything else into perspective' - Doe Zantamata

The quote by T.S. Elliot about it being the journey rather than the destination that matters is more appropriate to retirement than you might think. Think of it as a long journey of exploration and discovery. But take your time and prepare for it as far in advance as you can. I wouldn't advise you to just hand in the minimum notice period to your employer. If you can, it's much better to ease yourself out of work and into retirement gently. Even alcoholics and drug addicts are weaned off their addictions. Don't go cold turkey. Give at least one year's notice and if your employer is willing to reduce the days you work from 4 to 3 to 2 over a period of 12 months if you can. Having Mondays and Fridays off is a good lead into retirement. It also gives your employer more time to recruit a replacement and for you to hand over responsibilities, train your replacement so you might be in a better negotiating position if you provide a one year notice period. My own employer incentivised this approach by offering an additional 4 weeks annual leave for 12 months notice of retirement. Use your annual leave, buy days off and any additional days off you might be fortunate enough to get for giving a long notice period to reduce your working week. This will avoid the dilemma of waking up one Monday morning and wondering what you're going to do now with no job to go to. I have seen people still talking about work at their retirement parties which clearly is a sign they weren't ready to leave. 12 months working on a reduced working week will allow you to phase yourself out of a work mindset and into a retirement mindset. Reducing your working week and potentially your salary to the equivalent of your retirement income might also make the financial transition easier too. Also try to avoid taking long holidays during your final year at work. You'll be having a very long break from work soon enough!

A word of caution here! What you definitely don't want to do is cut back your working week and keep on doing the same job with the same responsibilities. Cramming five days of work into a three or four day week and getting paid for a three or four day week is not a good idea. This happened to me for the first 9 months of my 12 month retirement notice. I did 'make amends' for this in my final three months though once my replacement had been appointed to take over from me. So make sure you agree with your employer exactly what they expect of you during your reduced working week and what responsibilities and workload can be taken off you. Depending on the type of job you have, this might not be an issue. But be careful, especially if there is likely to be a backlog of work for you to come back to after your long weekends. If you have a managerial or an office based job you might end up having 100's of unanswered emails waiting for you and you will be playing catch up every week and working longer hours during your shortened working week. Also make sure your out of office message redirects emails to your line manager or a nominated colleague to deal with in your absence.

You are also likely to have been working to a set work routine for the last 35 to 45 years. Getting out of bed, travelling to work, doing your shift, travelling back home, etc. Retiring from work will free up both your travelling time and time spent at work obviously and for me this meant about 50 hours per week on average. So it does make sense to plan a gradual transition from a full time job and daily commute into what will be a 'job and commute free retirement'. Psychologically and physiologically our bodies and minds like routine and schedules so take time and make plans to modify your routines and schedules over the last year of full time employment. I discuss this more in Step 7 - Create a New Routine.

I first started thinking seriously about retirement around the age of 50 and decided that I wanted to retire at 55. Whilst and the next 3 years couldn't come quickly enough, with about 2 years to go I was beginning to get cold feet. Of course that was 2020 and we had just entered a global pandemic so everyone's plans were on hold pretty much. I had planned to give my retirement notice on my 54th birthday but as it turned out I procrastinated for another seven months because of the Pandemic before I finally gave my retirement notice to my manager. I also got agreement that I could reduce my working week from 4 to 3 to 2 days over the following 12 months.

But within just a few days of handing in my notice I had begun to feel some buyers' regret and was wondering if I'd done the right thing, despite having just spent the last 4 years thinking things through. Happy to report it didn't take me too long to get through this phase and I soon came to terms with the new mindset I had to adopt. My focus now was going to be on my exit strategy out of my life of work and my entry strategy into my new life of retirement. Now I had finally made my decision about what I was doing and I had a date to aim for, I felt both relaxed and excited about the future. I had agreed with my line manager that I would spend my final year completing the current projects I was involved in, I would not take on any new projects or responsibilities and I would gradually hand over my responsibilities to my replacement and step back from my day to day responsibilities. However, as I said it took them 9 months to appoint someone to replace me and this did make things quite stressful, especially when I was down to working a 3 day week. Fortunately my replacement was someone I liked and knew very well, who had worked in the company in a similar role to me for a number of years so it made for an easier handover and transition, which to a certain extent made up for the pressures of the previous 9 months.

If you do manage to take additional time off work during your final year, be careful not to rush into taking on too many out of work commitments like I did. Before I had retired I had taken on 4 volunteering roles, started writing this book and changed and changed my exercise routine from cycling 2 days per week to cycling, swimming and lifting weights 5 days a week. The result being, I spread myself very thinly across everything I was doing and didn't have much time left to do much else. I also suffered a painful back and chest injury from exercising when I was over tired which took me out for about 6 weeks where the only exercise I could do was on my indoor bike. There will be plenty of time to take on new hobbies, volunteering roles and exercise if that is what you want to do so there's no need to rush it. Take your time to adjust into your new lifestyle. Give yourself time to think. Go for some long walks in the fresh air and sunshine. Listen to your favourite music. Slowing things down also means giving yourself more time to do the simple or routine things in life like more time in bed, shopping, preparing and eating meals, spending time with friends and family, exercising or even household chores and DIY. When you are working many of these things can get rushed if you are time pressed with work commitments. This transition should be a period of reflection and thought about your future so take your time and enjoy it.

It's also good to take more time doing the things you enjoy. I find taking a bit more time allows me to focus on the present, on what I am doing in the moment or just soaking up what's happening around me. It's enjoyable to feel a part of something. Again I'm not naturally a sociable person but I do like to feel being part of a community, part of society. Since retiring I have also found greater pleasures in simple things like walking the dog. I started noticing more about the town I live in. The architectural beauty of some of the old sandstone buildings, hotels, the bridges, the train station, the natural beauty of the river, the trees, the parks or even just the presence of other people, the nod to other dog walkers, the bustle of town centre shoppers. Things I never really paid attention to in the past. When I was working, a dog walk was a functional activity. It was exercise for both myself and the dog obviously but it was just a walk. I would have walked anywhere and wouldn't be paying too much attention to the environment around me. I would be thinking about what I needed to do when I got home or at work the next day. Now I like to walk for the sake of walking. It's an interesting and enjoyable experience for me now.

Dan McDermott has an interesting blog at retiretbydegrees.com and discusses taking a slow phased approach into retirement. He says, 'It's more beneficial to retire gradually over many years, not abruptly in a single day. My goal is to explore planning for a staged retirement. Ratcheting down a full commitment to work and plan for retirement by setting goals, talking to others about their experience and committing to timelines. Experience it by starting to explore other areas of interest that may have been dormant for some time, travel, learning, etc. which if you keep putting off you may someday find you have very little time left to embrace them'.

Step 6 - Pursuing Meaningful Things

'It is in responsibility that most people find the meaning that sustains them through life. It is not in happiness. It is not in impulsive pleasure. It is a luxury to pursue what makes you happy. It is a moral obligation to pursue what you find meaningful' - Jordan Peterson.

For me personally this is one of the most important steps to take in retirement. My father paid me an unintentional compliment, I think, when I was around the age of 7 or 8 when I was playing on the floor with some bits of old lego he had recovered from other street urchins during his rag and bone phase. Observing me closely I overheard him saying to my mother, 'he would have no problem doing a stretch'. If you don't know what this means, it's slang for spending some time at Her Majesty's pleasure. I wasn't old enough to understand what he meant at the time but it stuck with me and on reflection I think he was observing that I always kept myself busy and never really complained about getting bored despite us having very little money for toys or activities. An observation, I am happy to report, I have thus far still managed to uphold and my late fathers hypothesis remains untested. If you are easily bored and you don't already have meaningful things to do to fill the gap in your life that retirement will bring then you are probably most likely not yet ready to retire. Maybe you think not liking your job is a sufficient reason for you to retire but you might dislike the extra time that not working will bring you even more if you don't have things to do with it. Especially if you plan on retiring early.

So what will you do with your time? It would be easy to surrender much of it to passive armchair activities like Social Media, reading newspapers, magazines, watching TV, subscription channels, box sets, sports channels, etc. Then of course there are the domestic activities like cooking, cleaning, shopping, laundry, chauffeuring children, etc that could take up even more of your time. Also don't underestimate other people becoming more demanding of your time when they find out you've retired. Oh you're retired, you've got time on your hands, can you help me with.... Although these activities are just part and parcel of everyone's life and they will continue in retirement, it's important not to let them expand too much and entirely fill that gap that retirement will bring.

So what type of things are meaningful to you? What things give you a sense of purpose? In Step 1 'Why Retire', I asked you to make a list of the things you would miss the most about your work and to think about replacements for them. For me these were Financial Security covered, Friendship & Camaraderie and Purpose, Meaning and Recognition.

What Inspires You

What things give your life value, meaning and purpose? Here are some examples of things that might inspire or motivate you as well as suggested activities that could fill that gap that leaving work life will bring. If any of these activities inspire or motivate you then give some thought as to how you can achieve them in your retirement.

What Inspires or Motivates You?	What You Can Do
Personal Goals & Development	Education, sport, learning new skills, taking on new challenges
Inventing or Creating New Things	Art, writing, painting, music
Helping Other People	Charity work, volunteering, fundraising, improving things for the people around you
Wealth & Security	Building financial wealth and security for you and your family
Relationship Building	Maintaining existing and building new friendships
Freedom	Able to decide what, when and how you do things

Or maybe you already have some hobbies, social activities, interests and responsibilities you can spend more time on or you could explore some new activities to see what sparks your interest. You've got time on your hands that you've never had before. There are probably a few things you maybe even only want to do once. Just for the experience. Or maybe you can only afford to do it once! Like flying first class or parachuting out of an aeroplane for example - probably not on the same flight though! Other activities you try might become lifelong passions. I talk about retirement bucket lists in Step 12 so this might give you further food for thought.

Replace your career goals with personal goals. Your job will have provided you with both physical, mental challenges and goals to achieve and aim for and it's important to find equally challenging goals in your retirement. I talk more about setting personal goals in Steps 8&9 for maintaining your physical and mental health and wellbeing. There are plenty of challenges out there - learning a new language, playing a musical instrument, studying for an academic qualification, researching a subject of interest, reading books, watching documentaries, educational boxsets, you-tube videos, podcasts, etc. on virtually anything you can think of. Learning doesn't stop in retirement. In fact it should give you more time to flourish in this area. There are unlimited resources including public libraries, online and on campus college courses and online learning platforms like Wondrium or u3a.org.uk - a UK-wide collection of 1000+ charities that provide the opportunity for those no longer in work to come together and learn for fun.

It might be useful to create a list of short, medium and long term goals. These could be a mixture of personal, health, family, relationship, social, financial, educational, societal and charitable goals. Update your list and tick things off as you have done them and add new ones to replace them. Revisit your list every few months or whenever you think is appropriate. Remember these are your goals. You get to decide what they are and what success means, not your employer and no-one is measuring except you.

Here are some suggestions to get you started:

Short Term

- Sort out your pensions and retirement finances
- Update your Will and Power of Attorney Documents
- Expand or start an exercise regime
- Find a new subject to study
- Find some charities and donate some of your time
- Make contact with old friends
- Join a club and make new friends

Medium Term

- Learn to draw, paint or play a musical instrument
- Write a book
- Travel to countries you've never been to before
- Learn to speak a different language
- Support your children/grandchildren through College/University

Long Term

- Move or downsize your house, follow your children
- Help your children/grandchildren to get on the housing ladder
- Live abroad for a few months each year

Write - Starting with Your Own Story

'Writing is thinking formalised. You gain the ability to think by first learning to write very, very carefully. Then, when you can write effectively, you can do anything you want, and no one will stop you. If you can think, and speak, and write, you are absolutely deadly' - Jordan Peterson

You know the old saying, 'everyone has at least one good book in them'. So have a go and write one. Start with writing your own story. Your memoirs might never get published but your family at least will probably enjoy reading them. You don't need to write down all of the darkest secrets that might hurt family members or have you spend the rest of your retirement in prison, but do tell the truth - or at least don't tell lies. Writing about your life in a chronological order can be a cathartic process. It will give you a chance to reconcile any unresolved issues, regrets, grudges, resentments, unmade apologies, etc. Jordan Peterson has an online course called 'The Self Authoring Program' that gets you to write about your past, present and future that I would recommend. Once you've written your own story you can offer to write other people's stories. There is a market out there now for biography writing.

You could also write about nonfiction topics of interest. If you have become an expert through your work or through hobbies then write about those. As I said, I could not find too much out there on retirement planning (apart from the financial side of things) which was the main driver for me writing this. I also wanted to write about my experiences as I was having them. Or if you are taking up a new hobby, sport or studying a new subject that interests you then you could write about these. Or maybe you could write a daily blog, journal or newsletter on a social media site or on Substack your thoughts and observations of current affairs topics of interest. Or you could offer to write articles for any clubs or societies you are involved with.

See one, do one, teach one is a tip I would offer to young trainees at work when it came to learning new skills but now I would add 'write things down' if you want to become an expert in something. I also believe writing down what you have seen, experienced or read helps to consolidate your understanding as well as committing things to memory. I initially just write down my thoughts and ideas, not worrying too much about the spelling, grammar or order of paragraphs or chapters even. I then come back to it at a later stage to tidy things up and clarify what I'm trying to say, fill any gaps and remove content that doesn't make sense. If nothing else it will give you something to read in your later years that you might have forgotten about had you not written it down. It also gives you something to leave as a legacy and for family members to read too.

Become a Minimalist

In his 1979 speech 'Crisis of Confidence', President Jimmy Carter said, 'Human identity is no longer defined by what one does, but by what one owns. But we've discovered that owning things and consuming things does not satisfy our longing for meaning'. Joshua Field Milburn and Ryan Nicodemus' book, 'Love People not Things: Because the Opposite Never Works' covers the subject of Minimalism. They also have a Netflix documentary called 'Minimalism' where they discuss why so many of us wrongly try to find meaning and a sense of identity from what we own rather than from what we do and how we can go about reversing this situation. 'Minimalism is the thing that gets us past the (material) things in our lives so we can make room for life's important things - which aren't things at all. Minimalism itself is not a new idea: the concept dates back to the Stoics. What's new is the problem: never before have people been more seduced by materialism, and never before have people been so willing to forsake loved ones to acquire heaps of meaningless stuff. By removing the physical distractions around us we are able to look inside ourselves and begin the mental, emotional, psychological and spiritual process of decluttering'. They also have a Podcast and a free ebook called '16 Rules for Living with Less'.

You can start by sorting out your personal possessions. I started in my attic, moved to my wardrobe, then the garage and finally the kitchen. I had notes from University that were 35 years old, 100's of vinyl records, CDs, DVD's and yet no longer actually owned a record player, CD or DVD player with which to play any of them. Although I had actually kept the original boxes and packaging for this equipment. Add to this, the books, clothes, sports equipment, 4 bikes (all for different types of cycling of course), camping equipment, tools, old tins of paint and their associated stirring sticks, garden tools (I don't have any grass, trees or plants. In the kitchen of course we had many unmatching dinner sets, cups, glasses and cutlery. Our novelty mug collection alone took up a full shelf. Not to mention the out of date food and cooking ingredients. Particularly stuff we bought during lockdown to bake with. I gave most of my clutter to local charity shops, some to the local waste tip and some I sold on ebay. A word of caution here. There might be a temptation to fill the empty spaces you've created with new clutter with the money you have made selling your old clutter.

Step 7 - Create a New Routine

'As humans, our bodies and more to the point, our minds, crave the comfort and mindlessness that routine offers. Routine requires very little conscious thought, freeing our brain to focus on more complex tasks. This makes everyday tasks, like commuting, brushing our teeth, taking a shower, and so on, second nature. When we aren't thinking about those necessities, we can pay more attention to other parts of our lives. If we've learned anything from the pandemic, the unexpected can happen, and it can cause anxiety. Having a routine will lower your anxiety because there's no conscious thought in the everyday details of life' - Samantha Dutton, PhD, at the University of Phoenix from an article in realsimple.com by Lindsay Tigar.

We can all agree that routine is hugely important for children. A bedtime routine is associated with increased family functioning and improved sleep habits. Family routines have been linked to the development of social skills and academic success and adherence to family routines has been identified as important for family resilience during times of crisis. However, the importance of routine is not unique to children. Observational research indicates that individuals in good health also engage in routine healthy behaviours. For example, those successful at maintaining weight loss often eat the same foods, engage in consistent exercise, and do not skip meals.

Routines will help you to create healthy habits and reduce stress levels. When you are organised and have a set routine, you know what to expect. This takes the anxiety out of thinking about what is coming next. Having days with nothing planned in front of you could lead to boredom, anxiety, and ultimately depression. Routines can liberate your mental health and bring psychological benefits including alleviating symptoms of mental disorders and insomnia. Think of them as habits. Create good ones and avoid bad ones.

How many hours do (or did) you spend on an average week at work, including your commute? For me it was about 50 hours. Okay that's the time you'll have back in your life to rebuild a new routine with. It doesn't need to be regimented as tightly as it might have been at work but it is important to have a schedule, even if it's a loose one. Whilst waking up in the morning and wondering what you're going to be doing with your day at weekends or on holiday might have been a luxury, it could soon become a source of stress, depression and anxiety in retirement if you do not have a new routine to replace your old one. The anxiety of having too few choices of what to do can be just as bad as having too many choices. Getting up and going to bed, eating meals and exercising at regular times, household chores, shopping, hobbies, volunteering, socialising with friends and family, even sitting down to relax in the evenings are the kind of things to incorporate into your new daily routine.

So create a new routine for your typical day/week and split it up and decide what parts of the day you're going to spend doing what. I still treat my weekdays differently to my weekends. I prefer my weekdays to be more structured so that I know what I'm doing from one day to the next. Weekdays are also the days your children/partner are likely to be at school, college or work so you might end up spending a fair bit of it on your own so it's a good thing to have a structure and routine to these days to avoid boredom and anxiety. The weekends I tend not to structure so much and leave them open to whatever events or opportunities come my way. I usually wake up around 7am, about an hour later than when I was working, then spend half an hour catching up on news, social media, emails, etc on my phone. I'll then get up, have breakfast, see my son out to school and then exercise for about 60 minutes. I'll then maybe spend some time on household chores, shopping, dog walking etc. After lunch I'll spend time on personal projects such as writing, charity work, studying, reading or whatever else I have on the go at the time. I'll usually always be listening to something on the radio or a podcast or music if I'm doing things on my own during the day. When the family comes home in the evening I'll make dinner and by this point in the day I'm back to where I was before retirement. I avoid watching any TV before 6pm unless it's a live sporting event or a news programme I'm interested in. Same rule for drinking alcohol and usually only at weekends for that.

You can also think about weekly, monthly or even annual routines. So you might want to keep a diary, a wall calendar or use a mobile phone app for recording events, social activities, lunch dates, nights out at the cinema or theatre, nights out with friends & relatives, sporting events, holidays, birthdays, anniversaries, etc. Having things planned, written down and diarised all gives you things to look forward to in the future. But don't be a slave to your routine and don't let it stifle spontaneity or stop you from taking opportunities that come your way. Look at it as something to fall back on if there aren't other matters more deserving of your time.

Oliver Burkeman's book, 4000 Weeks - Time and how to Use it talks about 'how we are obsessed with our ever lengthening to-do lists, overfilled inboxes, the struggle against distraction and the sense that our attention spans are shrivelling and yet were rarely make the connection between our daily struggle against time and the ultimate time management problem: how to use our ridiculously brief time on the planet, amounting to about 4000 weeks'. His philosophical look at how we manage our time dispels the popular time management, productivity and efficiency techniques and explains that no matter how hard we try we will never have enough time to do what we think needs to get done. In fact the harder we try to get more things done on our to-do lists, it only ends up in more things being added to it. Burkeman offers suggestions for constructing a meaningful life by embracing rather than denying our limitations. One of the things I learnt from reading the book was the advice to limit the number of new projects you take on at any one time and to try focusing on only one project at a time. I took on far too many volunteering roles leading into retirement and at the same time I was trying to write this book and was building up my exercise routine as well as adapting to a new routine in a life without work. When you're working it's probably easier to run with multiple tasks or projects as you're likely to have a high level of competence in what you're doing but when you retire you're learning new skills so perhaps so you'll be less competent and more prone to anxiety from doing too many new things at the same time. So be conscious of this. Definitely one for your retirement reading list I would suggest.

Step 8 - Looking after your Physical Health

'It is a shame for a man to grow old without seeing the beauty and strength of which his body is capable' - Socrates.

There is a common myth that retirement can be detrimental to your health however a study by Tilburg University concluded, 'The effect that health has on the retirement decision has long been studied. We examined the reverse relationship, whether retirement has a direct impact on later-life health. We found no negative effects of early retirement on men's health and if anything, a temporary increase in self-reported health and improvements in health of highly educated workers`.

Peter Attia's book *Outlive: The Science and Art of Longevity* offers a comprehensive guide to extending both lifespan and healthspan—the quality of one's life. Attia identifies the "Four Horsemen" of aging: heart disease, cancer, neurodegenerative diseases, and type 2 diabetes. He advocates for a proactive approach to mitigate these risks through lifestyle modifications in five key areas: exercise, nutrition, sleep, emotional health, and the strategic use of supplements or medications:

Exercise: Attia emphasizes that exercise is the most potent tool for longevity. He recommends incorporating Zone 2 training (steady-state cardio) for mitochondrial efficiency, VO_2 max training to enhance cardiovascular fitness, and strength training to maintain muscle mass and functional independence. Additionally, he highlights the importance of stability and balance exercises to prevent falls and injuries, especially in older age.

Nutrition: Rather than endorsing specific diets, Attia focuses on nutritional biochemistry. He advises adequate protein intake (at least 0.8 grams per kilogram of body weight), minimizing processed foods and added sugars, and prioritizing monounsaturated fats found in olive oil, avocados, and nuts. Monitoring glucose levels is also recommended to prevent metabolic dysfunction.

Sleep: Quality sleep is deemed crucial for overall health. Attia suggests creating a dark, cool sleeping environment, avoiding alcohol and late meals, establishing consistent sleep and wake times, and aiming for at least eight hours of sleep opportunity each night.

Emotional Health: Attia underscores the significance of emotional well-being, advocating for the cultivation of meaningful relationships, stress management practices, and, when necessary, professional therapy. He posits that longevity is meaningless without quality of life, which is heavily influenced by emotional health.

By addressing these domains, Attia provides a strategic framework aimed at not only prolonging life but also enhancing its quality, effectively confronting the primary chronic diseases associated with aging.

Benefits of Exercise

The benefits of physical exercise (at any age) are already well documented. Current guidelines from health professionals say that engaging in around 150 minutes of moderate intensity activity or 75 minutes of vigorous intensity activity per week decreases the risk of mortality by 27%. Vigorous activity makes you breathe hard and fast, making it difficult to say more than a few words without pausing. This might include running, cycling, swimming and sports such as football and rugby. Moderate activity makes you breathe faster, but you will still be able to talk. Examples might include playing golf, brisk walking, hiking, climbing a flight of stairs or pushing a lawn mower.

Physical activity reduces many major mortality risk factors including arterial hypertension, type 2 diabetes, dyslipidemia, coronary heart disease, stroke and cancer. Exercise also improves mental health by reducing anxiety, depression & negative mood as well as improving cognitive function and has also been found to alleviate symptoms such as low self-esteem and social withdrawal. Exercise also improves your sleep quality.

Before I retired, my only fitness activity had essentially been only road cycling. I would routinely cycle on 4 days/week averaging about 100 miles a week. I would cycle on 2 days at lunchtimes at work and then do 2 longer rides on the weekends and would occasionally also cycle the 30 miles to or from work. I mostly cycled on my own and listened to music, news or podcasts and I would do this in all kinds of weather. Only ice or snow on the ground would stop me from going out and even then I would sometimes give it a go. All of this would mean I was cycling on average around 5 to 6 hours per week. Plus another 4 hours for getting myself and the bike prepped and cleaned at the start and end of the rides. Not to mention the time recovery after 3 hour long cycle runs on the weekends where my activities were usually limited to lying on the sofa (often watching cycling on the TV). So I was spending a fair bit of time on only doing one type of exercise and I really wasn't fit for any other sports other than cycling. I was quite thin with fairly low muscle mass and strength but I did have good cardio fitness. I was brought to my senses in my late 40's when out cycling one lunchtime at work in the rain when the front wheel slid from under me as I was going down a winding narrow single track road. My Fitbit recorded that (my chest) hit the tarmac at 26 mph. I remembered the tip not to put my hand out to save myself and avoided a broken collar bone. Interestingly, fitness monitors are commonly used these days to help determine the cause of death of their wearers! I called my office and asked them to call me an ambulance. By the time it arrived I was so cold it took about half an hour before they could get a needle into my arm to give me painkillers before embarking on a bumpy ride to the hospital. I was lucky to have only suffered soft tissue damage to my ribs however I'll not forget the pain and the length of time it took to make a full recovery. I was off the bike for about 6 months.

This experience however did give me the time to think about what I was trying to achieve with my fitness goals. I wasn't racing or competing, it wasn't even a social activity and the thing was, whilst I had reasonably good cardiovascular fitness, I was only really fit for cycling! I've spoken to other people who only ever swam or ran and again they too said the same thing, they were only fit for swimming or running. They, like me, struggled when it came to doing different sports or fitness activities. Whenever I tried running or swimming I very quickly got out of breath. Same for when I tried hiking and even worse when I tried playing tennis or basketball with my son. Whilst I had reasonably good aerobic fitness for cycling, the muscles I was using when I tried anything else just weren't up to the job. Just because you are fit for one type of exercise doesn't mean you will be fit for another. The lateral movements, strength, balance, flexibility, physical coordination and changes of speed you will need for playing tennis are completely different from swimming, running or cycling.

Functional Fitness

When you were younger you might have engaged in sports or physical activities for competitive or social reasons or even just to make yourself look and feel good. When you get older your exercise regime should be more aligned to support the type of lifestyle and activities you want to be doing and to allow you to live a healthy, happy and injury free retirement. This is commonly described as functional fitness. Functional fitness means doing movements that mimic everyday actions, incorporating multiple muscle groups at the same time. This builds strength, stability and mobility across the body, making us more efficient human beings not only inside the gym but outside as well.Functional fitness is useful for simple things in day to day life like running for a bus or a train, picking up or playing with your grandchildren, lifting heavy shopping bags, moving furniture around the house, lifting heavy suitcases into your car or into the overhead locker on a plane, digging the garden, mowing the lawn, painting a ceiling, climbing a ladder or washing the car even.

Functional fitness can be broken down into 6 different types of exercise but you can group them into 3 sub-groups; aerobic & anaerobic, muscle & strength and balance & flexibility. You can think of this combination of activities as a diversified fitness portfolio, except the difference with a fitness portfolio is that it's something you need to keep investing in to get continued benefit from it. Unlike a diversified financial portfolio where you would normally stop investing in it when you retire, if you stop investing in your fitness portfolio your physical assets are very soon going to depreciate and deteriorate. But you shouldn't wait until you retire to start preparing for your functional fitness routine any more than you would wait to retire to start building your financial portfolio.

Aerobic and Anaerobic Fitness

Aerobic means 'with air' and refers to the body producing energy with the use of oxygen. This typically involves any exercise that lasts longer than two minutes in duration. Continuous 'steady state' exercise is performed aerobically. This could be running, cycling, swimming at a steady pace. Anaerobic means 'without air' and refers to the body producing energy without oxygen. This typically involves short bursts of high intensity exercise such as sprinting, climbing a few flights of stairs or walking up a short steep hill or high intensity interval training - HIIT. But having good aerobic fitness doesn't necessarily mean you will have good anaerobic fitness. You need to practise both. HIIT can be done in short bursts of fast running, cycling or swimming so you can combine your aerobic and your anaerobic exercises at the same time. Aerobic fitness is useful if you're out on a long hike, walk or cycle with friends. Anaerobic fitness is useful for running for that bus or climbing the stairs if the lift is out of service. Aerobic and anaerobic fitness are both good for heart and circulatory health.

Balance

According to the authors of a study in the British Journal of Sports Medicine (in a Times article from June 2022), from your 50's onwards, if you can't stand on one leg, like a flamingo, without wobbling for at least 10 seconds then you are at almost twice the risk of dying within ten years than those who can hold a flamingo-like posture. In their 12-year study, researchers found participants inability to stand unsupported on one leg for ten seconds whilst resting their free foot on the back of the leg they are balancing on whilst staring forwards was associated with an 84% raised risk of death from any cause. Poor balance is a known side effect of underlying medical conditions including inner ear infections, hearing loss, Parkinson's, Alzheimer's, Stroke, reduced cognitive function and dementia. Research has indicated that whilst a lack of balance is rarely a cause of ill health it can be a strong marker for it. It is a general but reliable indicator of physical decline and some deterioration in balance is inevitable as we get older. Whilst we can't avoid it, we can slow the deterioration by building up to doing 60 seconds of balancing on each leg three times daily. And once you've mastered that try doing it with your eyes closed. There's also evidence that doing these exercises improves hip bone density of people in their seventies, reducing the risk of a fracture if you do fall.

Flexibility

Maintaining flexibility not only improves your performance in daily activities but also decreases your risk of injury, decreases pain in your upper back, helps relieve and prevent lower back pain, improves your workouts due to better muscular performance, improves posture and helps you keep a more youthful appearance by reducing shuffling or hunching over.

Muscle Mass and Strength

Age-related muscle loss is a natural part of ageing. After age 30, you begin to lose as much as 3% to 5% per decade. Most men will lose about 30% of their muscle mass during their lifetimes. Lifting weights or resistance training are the best exercises for retaining and building muscle mass and strength. Lifting heavier weights whilst doing lower repetitions is good for building muscle strength and lifting lighter weights whilst doing higher repetitions is good for building muscle mass. You can do simple things at home like push ups, sit ups, squats and lunges using your own body weight as resistance. You can increase resistance by investing in some basic kit for your home like dumbbells, kettlebells, resistance bands and an exercise mat or you can join a local gym if you prefer the social aspect to fitness training.

Motivation

Starting a new exercise regime is easier at the beginning when you have the motivation and are keen to get started. The initial benefits you gain from exercise will also help drive that motivation further but you might come to a plateau as the law of diminishing returns kicks in as even smaller gains become harder to achieve. Gyms are always at their busiest in January as people make new year resolutions to get fit and then attendances gradually decline over the year as they lose motivation or find they no longer enjoy what it is they are doing. So it's important to find out what keeps you motivated. Dr Jennifer Heisz' book, 'Move the Body, Heal the Mind - Overcome Anxiety Depression, Dementia and Improve Focus', gives some good advice on exercise motivation including swilling a sugary drinks in your mouth, bargaining with yourself on an easy workout if you're tired, listening to music, focusing on your breathing, listening to your body clock and exercising with friends.

What Do I Do Now

I always exercise in the mornings, straight after breakfast usually. As the day goes on my energy and motivation levels decline. Peter Attia's 'Outlive' has a rule of thumb for exercise where you should allocate 50% of your weekly available time to strength and stability training and 50% to cardio training. For cardio training you should split the time 80/20 between zone 2 and zone 5 heart training. I currently exercise for 60 minutes a day, 5 days a week and I do both cardio and weights on every day. On 4 of the 5 days I will do 30 minutes of cardio on an indoor bike, step or elliptical machines in zone 2 heart rate for cardio and for the second 30 minutes of these sessions I lift weights for strength and stability. On the 5th day I will do a 40 minute session of VO2 Max training on an indoor bike. This consists of an 8 minute warm up in zone 1 followed by four sets of 4 minutes in zone 5 followed by four minutes in zone 1. I then do weights for the final 20 minutes of this session. I alternate my workouts between the gym and home where I have an indoor bike and a small set of dumbbells and kettlebells. I will very occasionally go for outdoor bike rides and I have my daily 30 minute dog walks so I have a variety of options for exercising, covering the different areas for functional fitness and with enough variety to keep myself motivated. I've really enjoyed having the extra time in retirement to develop my exercise routine and it's certainly a lot better for me than just cycling 100's of miles on the roads every month which I have now greatly reduced, mainly due to a few near misses I have had with motorists getting a bit too close on country roads.

So create your own diversified fitness routine that will give you the functional fitness for the type of retirement you want to live. If you're not used to doing regular exercise then remember to build it up gradually. Find out which time of day is best for you and stick with it. Take it easy to begin with, try different activities to find out what you enjoy. You can do it with your partner or friends and make it a social activity and have alternatives to fall back on in case of bad weather or injuries. And if you do get injuries it's not the end of the world. They will heal given time but do try to do something to keep moving even when injured. Find a good sports physio, they're worth their weight in gold. Stretching the injured muscles works for me as do gel ice packs for reducing pain and inflammation. I have kept one in my freezer for over 10 years now.

NHS or Private Healthcare

The British Medical Association stated in May 2022 - 'It will take years to clear the backlog of patient treatment and appointments from the Covid 19 Pandemic. The ongoing need for stringent infection prevention control measures and workforce shortages means it will take even longer to work through as demand continues to rise. The number of people on NHS waiting lists for consultant-led elective care rose from 4.2 Million in March 2020 to 6.18 Million in February 2022. The total number of patients waiting over 18 weeks for treatment now exceeds 2 million, whilst the number of patients waiting over one year for treatment stands at almost 300,000. This is 186 times the number waiting over a year pre-pandemic in February 2020. Between April 2020 and February 2022, compared to pre-COVID averages, there were 4.5 million fewer elective procedures and 31.4 million fewer outpatient attendances. This is storing up greater problems for the future. These backlogs are likely to result in worsened conditions down the line, leading to greater demand on health services'.

According to the ONS, healthcare expenditure in the UK in 2018 was £214.4 billion, equating to £3,227 per person, accounting for 10% of gross domestic product (GDP). Although nearly three-quarters (73%) consider the NHS to be one of the UK's greatest achievements, more than four in ten believe the NHS will not survive in its current form to the end of the current decade.

So it's clear there are problems in the NHS that are going to take some time to put right, if that's even possible, but in the meantime are you prepared to wait and endure any ongoing medical issues or are you prepared to go private. According to finder.com the average premium for UK private health insurance is £1,435 per year (you can get it much cheaper than this if you increase your excess and exclude pre-existing conditions). Over half (53%) of the UK population admitted they would pay for private healthcare treatment and 13% of UK consumers claim to belong to a Private Medical Insurance scheme.

I had private healthcare with my employer for 16 years and used it for conditions I would almost certainly never have received treatment for on the NHS. After suffering in silence for a number of years with shoulder pain I remembered I had private health care that I had never used before and so contacted my insurer who arranged an appointment for me with an orthopaedic consultant in Glasgow. Within the space of 10 minutes of being in his office he had examined me, diagnosed the issue and booked me in for an operation 7 days later. It took 3 months of post op physio before I had fully recovered and my shoulder has been fine since. A few years later I had a similar operation on my other shoulder. I appreciate there are many people out there with much worse conditions than I had but I suppose at the end of the day it's about how much you value your health and wellbeing. If you have medical issues you believe are unlikely to get treated on the NHS or you are having to wait years on a waiting list and you can afford to go private then why not. You can consider if you want to pay for this through an insurance policy or on a pay as you go basis. Something else to factor into your retirement expenses. Under your 'Needs' I would suggest.

Measure your Vitals

Body Mass Index - The Body Mass Index measurement uses your height and weight to work out if you're a healthy weight, underweight or overweight. Your BMI result is not the perfect measure of your overall health. It can't tell if you're carrying too much fat or you've got a lot of muscle, however you can use your BMI as a starting point for further discussion with your GP. Some points to note about the BMI are:

- Older adults can have a healthy BMI but still have too much fat. This is because older adults tend to have more body fat than younger adults.
- Women can have a healthy BMI but still have too much fat. This is because women tend to have more body fat than men with the same BMI.
- If you're from a black and ethnic minority group, you're at increased risk of type 2 diabetes with a BMI of 23 or more.
- An athletic adult with a lot of muscle may have a high BMI but not be overweight. This is because BMI can't tell the difference between fat and muscle.

Taking these limitations into account, the BMI is a relatively straightforward and convenient way of initially assessing your weight. I have included a link to the NHS BMI calculator in the Resources section. You input your weight, height, age, sex and ethnic group and activity level and it will give you the healthy weight range for your height. A healthy adult BMI is between 18.5 kg/m2 to 24.9 kg/m2.

You can also buy relatively inexpensive body fat scales which use a method known as bioelectrical impedance analysis (BIA), which sends a weak electric current through your body to determine your body composition including body mass index, fat free body weight, bone mass, muscle mass as well as percentages of - body fat, subcutaneous fat, visceral fat, body water, body water as well as your body's metabolic age.

Waist Measurement - Whilst measuring body mass index (BMI) is useful, it doesn't take into account excess weight around the abdomen. Measuring your waist is a good way to check you're not carrying too much fat around your stomach, which can raise your risk of heart disease, type 2 diabetes and stroke. You can have a healthy BMI and still have excess fat around the waist meaning you're still at risk of developing these conditions. To measure your waist, find the bottom of your ribs and top of your hips, wrap a tape measure around your waist midway between these points, breathing out naturally before taking the measurement. According to the NHS and regardless of your height or BMI, you should try to lose weight if your waist is over 94cm (37ins) for men and 80cm (31.5ins) for women. You're at very high risk and should contact a GP if your waist is 102cm (40ins) or more for men and 88cm (34ins) or more for women.
The National Institute for Care and Excellence recommends that an adult's waist should be less than half their height to reduce health risks.

Blood Pressure - Blood pressure is recorded with 2 numbers. The systolic pressure (higher number) is the force at which your heart pumps blood around your body. The diastolic pressure (lower number) is the resistance to the blood flow in the blood vessels. They're both measured in millimetres of mercury (mmHg). As a general guide normal blood pressure is usually considered to be between 90/60mmHg and 120/80mmHg. High blood pressure is considered to be 140/90mmHg or higher (or 150/90mmHg or higher if you're over the age of 80). Blood pressure readings between 120/80mmHg and 140/90mmHg could mean you're at risk of developing high blood pressure if you do not take steps to keep it under control. Everyone's blood pressure will be slightly different. What's considered low or high for you may be normal for someone else. You can also pick up a blood pressure monitor fairly cheaply these days.

Fitness Trackers - You might also want to invest in a smartwatch. You can link these to an app on your phone and track all your vital stats. I use a Fitbit but there are plenty of other brands out there. Again, a relatively small investment but they give you great information by tracking things like heart rate, steps walked, calories burnt, sleep quality, blood oxygen levels as well as exercise tracking, distance walked and time spent in fat burning, cardio and peak exercise zones. Resting heart rate is a good indicator of your general fitness level and it's interesting to track this and see it drop as your fitness level improves. You can also see it rise if you are unwell or if you have an illness, infection or even a hangover! Smart watches can also give you a readiness score that tells you when to take it easy and when to exercise depending on your recent activity, sleep and heart rate variability

Bad Habits

I'm not going to preach to you on the harmful effects of smoking, excessive alcohol consumption and poor dietary habits. I smoked in my 20's and gave it up because I developed asthma. Not being able to breathe made giving up smoking easy for me. I drank alcohol as a way of relaxing and switching off from work at the end of the week, rarely on weeknights. I couldn't function if I was working the next day and drank the night before. Even one drink would disrupt my sleep and I'd be hungover and tired the next day. So having work the next day was a good motivator for not drinking the night before. One fear I had about retiring from a health perspective was that without the motivation of having to go to work the next day, I would start drinking more. That's where my morning exercise routine has helped. I know I have a workout to get up to do each morning. Not easy with a hangover. Like all things in life, moderation is the key. 14 units per week with 3 or 4 nights alcohol free is the current medical advice.

There are far too many topics on the subject of health, fitness, nutrition and wellbeing to cover in a book on retirement planning and again as I said at the start of the book, I am not an expert in this area. I am only sharing my own thoughts, experiences and what I have researched. I have included some links and references to some of the issues discussed in Step 8 in the Resources section.

Step 9 - Looking After Your Mental Health

'About a third of my cases are suffering from no clinically definable neurosis, but from the senselessness and emptiness of their lives. This can be defined as the general neurosis of our times' - Carl Gustav Jung

Be Conscious of the Emotional Transition

It is important to understand there will be emotional ups and downs as you transition from your life in work to your new life in retirement. Feelings of apprehension, anxiety and even depression are not unusual. The emotional transition of retiring is not dissimilar to any other significant change we experience in life such as marriage, divorce, redundancy, serious illness, injuries or even the death of a loved one. Whilst many of these matters have been professionally studied and analysed to a large degree, the emotional and psychological impacts of retirement have not seen similar attention, until recently. The Kübler-Ross model has been extensively used by psychologists and organisations to help people understand their reactions and emotions to significant change or loss. The model holds true not only for someone going through a traumatic experience but also in going through retirement too.

So it is important to recognise that your emotions will change as you go through a process not dissimilar to that of grieving when you stop working and transition into retirement. There might be an initial feeling of elation when you stop working and you are looking forward to the next chapter in your life and what that will bring. This might be followed by a period of deflation as you no longer have your work routine and meaningful things to do. But then you will begin to adapt and adjust to a new routine with different people and doing different things. And as you experiment with new activities and take on new responsibilities and develop new relationships you begin to feel the positive emotions grow again. You begin to feel more in control, you're making decisions about how you will progress and integrate your new activities, responsibilities, routines and relationships into your life. Imagine it as an emotional rollercoaster where you ascend to an initial peak and then freefall for a bit before rapidly ascending to a point higher than from where you began. But it does take time and patience and some will transition through it faster than others. And you might even find yourself going backwards at some point. But what is important is to recognise that you are going through a transition and realise that you will get through it and adapt to your new life in retirement. But it's up to you to make sure the change is a positive one.

There's a great little TEDx Talk on YouTube by a Dr. Riley Moynes who talks about going through 4 distinct phases of retirement that I've linked to in the Resources. Phase 1 is the vacation stage which lasts about a year where your emotions are positive. Then the novelty wears off and you move into the negative Phase 2 where he talks about experiencing 5 losses including the loss of routine, sense of identity, relationships, sense of purpose and power. Phase 2 is also where you come face to face with the 3 D's - Depression, Divorce and Decline. Phase 3 is about experimenting with as many different things as you can to find things you enjoy doing and find the most meaningful. Phase 4 is the final stage where you recover the losses from phase 2, the phase to reinvent and rewire, to help others and as Dr. Riley says, 'squeeze all of the juice out of retirement'.

If you are feeling down or depressed then talk to your family and friends for support. Alternatively you can speak to charitable organisations such as ageuk.org.uk, thesilverline.org.uk, samaritans.org, findahelpline.com. All of whom have confidential helplines.

Sleep

'The best bridge between despair and hope is a good night's sleep' - Mathew Walker's book, Why we Sleep - Unlocking the Power of Sleep and Dreams, explains why more even than exercise, diet and wealth, science has shown that sleep is the most important factor to our physical and mental wellbeing. If you only read one book on improving your health and wellbeing or you have difficulty getting a good night's sleep or are keen to understand how you can improve the quality of your sleep, then please read Walker's book. He begins the book by saying that routinely sleeping less than 7 hours a night demolishes your immune system, more than doubles your risk of cancer, increases your risk of Alzheimer's and increases the likelihood of your coronary arteries becoming blocked and brittle. Setting you on a path towards cardiovascular disease, stroke and congestive heart failure. Even 1 week of inadequate sleep disrupts sugar levels so profoundly you would be classified as pre-diabetic. Alarmingly, vehicular accidents caused by drowsy driving exceed those caused by alcohol and drugs combined.

Walker's book goes on to talk in depth about the different stages of sleep and how they perform different but essential functions for maintaining good health and how sleep is the single most effective thing we can do to reset our brain and body health each day. Your body goes through several sleep cycles each night, on average 90 minutes each and within each cycle it alternates between REM sleep (rapid eye movement) and NREM sleep. NREM sleep has both light sleep and deep sleep. Periods of deep NREM sleep typically happen in the first half of the night and periods of REM in the second half.

REM sleep is typically associated with dreaming, where your brain becomes more active, your eyes move quickly, your heart rate rises and the muscles below your neck become inactive to prevent you from acting out your dreams in your sleep. REM is important for mood regulation, learning and memory. If you don't sleep the very first night after learning for example, you lose the chance to consolidate those memories, even if you get lots of catch-up sleep thereafter. In terms of memory then, sleep is not like the bank. You cannot accumulate a debt and hope to pay it off at a later point in time. Sleep for memory consolidation is an all-or-nothing event.

Deep sleep promotes physical recovery, some aspects of memory and learning and is also important for your immune system. During deep sleep your breathing rate slows, your heart beat is more regular, your muscles relax and you are likely to feel more refreshed in the morning if you've had some good deep sleep. As you get older the time spent in deep sleep reduces.

Fitness trackers are good for tracking your sleep patterns. They use a combination of body movement and heart rate variability and will show you the time spent in each phase of sleep as well as the time spent below your resting heart rate and restlessness levels, all useful indicators of your sleep quality.

On the plus side Walker also talks about the benefits of an afternoon nap and how this is the way that humans slept for many years. 'Hunter gatherer tribes in the Northern Kenya and the Kalahari desert who live without electricity and whose way of life has changed little over the past 1000's of years, sleep seven to 8 hours at night followed by a 30 to 60 minute nap in the afternoon. A study by Harvard University showed that people who engaged in these types of sleep patterns actually lived longer than those who did not'. So don't feel guilty if you do want to take that afternoon nap, but ideally no later than 3pm and no longer than 30 minutes as it will affect your sleep quality at night.

He ends the book with 12 tips for a healthy sleep including, 'having regular times for going to bed and getting up, exercising and getting sunlight 30 minutes of each per day, avoiding caffeine and nicotine (caffeine can take 8 hours to wear off), avoiding alcohol or large meals before bedtime, consulting with your doctor/pharmacist about any medication that might adversely affect your sleep, avoiding naps after 3pm, reading a book, taking a bath or listening to music before bed to relax and unwind, keeping your bedroom cool, dark and free of gadgets and finally not to lie in bed if you can't get to sleep but instead to get up and do something relaxing'.

As someone who suffers from poor sleep myself I would add a few of my own tips too:

1. Make sure that your mattress is both large enough (especially you are sharing it) and comfortable enough, is of good quality, not too soft and not too hard. I've moved from a hard to a soft mattress as I find it helps with aches and pains that come with age better.
2. If your partner is a snorer or a hugger and you're not then you might want to consider different beds (or different bedrooms even).

3. Wear an eye mask and ear plugs if you can't block out all of the light and noise in your bedroom.
4. And lastly there's an online app called Sleepio that offers CBT for insomnia that you can either pay to become a subscriber, or access for free via the NHS (in some parts of the UK). It's endorsed by the National Institute for Health and Care Excellence.

You spend a third of your life in bed so it's a worthwhile investment. If Goldilocks got it right then you can too!

Meditation and Mindfulness

'The habit of spending nearly every waking moment lost in thought leaves us at the mercy of whatever our thoughts happen to be. Meditation is a way of breaking this spell' - Sam Harris

The mental health charity mind.org.uk defines mindfulness as a technique that involves noticing what's happening in the present moment, without judgement. You might take notice and be aware of your mind, body or surroundings. The technique has roots in Buddhism and meditation. But you don't have to be spiritual, or have any particular beliefs, to try it. Mindfulness aims to help you become more self-aware, feel calmer and less stressed, feel more able to choose how to respond to your thoughts and feelings, cope with difficult or unhelpful thoughts and be kinder towards yourself. Many people find practising mindfulness helps them manage their day-to-day wellbeing, but it doesn't always work for everyone.

A technique that I use if I am feeling stressed, tense, anxious or can't get to sleep combines muscle relaxation and breathing methods. Sitting or lying down in a quiet space, close your eyes and begin to take deep breaths. After you have counted 10 breaths, begin the process of slowly tensioning and relaxing the muscles from your toes to your head, one group at a time. Starting with your toes and feet, gradually tension your muscles whilst slowly inhaling and counting to 5. When you reach the count of 5, hold your breath for 2 seconds and then gradually start releasing the tension and breathing out slowly whilst at the same time counting down from 5 to 1. When you reach 1 your tensed muscles should be fully relaxed and you should have fully exhaled your breath. Take another 1 or 2 slow deep breaths in and out then repeat the process, by gradually moving up your body one set of muscles at a time with your calf muscles, thighs, buttocks, stomach and lower back, hands, arms, neck, upper back back and shoulders and finishing off with your face and scalp muscles. Remember to take a full deep breath in and out between each set of muscles and at the end take 5 to 10 deep breaths whilst focusing on how relaxed your muscles are and how calm you are feeling.

Resilience

When we are faced with challenges and changes in life, our resilience helps us to deal with and manage those changes. It also helps us to adapt in times of adversity and to manage sources of stress and possible trauma without experiencing a significant impact on our wellbeing. Building physical and emotional resilience is important to ensure you have reserves to tap into or fall back on whenever you suffer a loss or a setback in life. Having good social connections and relationships, meaningful goals, hobbies, interests, physical activities, eating and sleeping well and limiting alcohol consumption are all important for building up resilience in retirement. The redcross.org.uk website has a good article on building resilience that I have linked to in the Resources section.

As I was writing this book I suffered a painful chest and back injury from overdoing it at the gym. Healing seemed to be very slow and every time I sneezed it felt like I was back to square one. I get restless and anxious if I am not doing some form of physical exercise and the first few weeks I did very little other than walking the dog and began to get down and depressed. I lost interest in doing anything productive or even having conversations. Fortunately I have an indoor exercise bike and I found I could do this without feeling too much pain so this gave me an outlet for exercising until I felt ready to go back to my normal activities. So having alternative options and activities to fall back on or to occupy yourself with when you suffer a setback is a good idea.

Sense of Identity

Having a sense of identity is important for your mental health in retirement. Who are you going to be when you walk out of the door or through the gates on your last day at work? What are you going to say when someone you know, or don't know, asks you what you are doing with yourself in retirement or what you do for a living? Are you just going to say, I'm retired? Or maybe you'll say I'm a retired - engineer, nurse, builder, lawyer, etc. But is that enough? Does that say who you are now or who you want to become? You will have built up a sense of identity from your job, your employer or profession that gave you a role in society that you had the right to be proud of. No longer being able to say you are doing this job will leave a gap to fill, so have a think about how you want to answer this question that will make you feel good about yourself. You don't have to justify yourself but people will be curious to know what you are doing in retirement. Especially the ones who are still working and maybe just a little bit envious! You could start by updating your social media status.

That should generate some conversations to get you started thinking before you have some of the face to face discussions. For the moment I've updated mine to: Cycling. Writing. Volunteering.

Loneliness

If you retire before your spouse/partner or if you are single, you might find yourself spending long periods on your own, so it's important to be mindful of the potentially detrimental mental health effects of loneliness in retirement. Whilst being alone at times might actually be a luxury, prolonged loneliness can have a detrimental effect on your mental health. So when your busy life at work stops and your free time increases significantly, you might find that being alone becomes a bigger part of your life.

According to the Campaign to End Loneliness, (in an article from wavelength.co.uk) over a million older people in the UK are chronically lonely. But this problem doesn't just impact the elderly. 53% of 18-34 year olds also struggle with loneliness. Human beings are social creatures and recent research has shown that feeling alone is not just upsetting, it's actually bad for your health. Over the last few years, scientists have been working to uncover the real impact that loneliness can have on our wellbeing. Studies have found that loneliness has been related to long term health issues. When someone is lonely their brain triggers a reaction that leads to a less active immune system and increased inflammation. Meaning people are less able to fight off viruses and have a slower recovery if they do get sick. Loneliness and social isolation are also risk factors for heart disease and stroke. Researchers have also found that people with fewer social connections have higher levels of the Coronary Heart Disease (CHD) and the stroke causing protein fibrinogen in their blood. Fibrinogen, which causes blood to clot, is released when our body is anticipating an injury – or when our brain triggers the fight or flight response. While this is essential when we cut ourselves, too much of it can lead to increased blood pressure and blocked arteries, which can ultimately lead to CHD and Stroke. All of these things combined mean that social isolation and loneliness are linked with a 30% higher risk of an early death. And while the discussion of loneliness tends to focus on elderly people, research has actually found that this risk is greater amongst people under the age of 65. Loneliness doesn't just damage physical health and shorten our life expectancy. A recent study has found that people who are lonely are more likely to later experience social anxiety, paranoia and depression, and that feelings of social anxiety are a predictor for future loneliness. Research has also shown that people with dementia are more likely to be lonely than those who don't and that lonely dementia sufferers experience a faster cognitive decline than those with more social connections.

Relationships

Like many people you will possibly spend more time with the people you work with than you do with your family and friends. But when you stop working it's likely that many of your work relationships will fade over time. So you will need to think about making new relationships, nurturing current ones and rekindling old ones in retirement. There might be some work friends you want to maintain so make sure you exchange personal contact details with them before you retire. You might also want to consider having a leaving party to celebrate your retirement and invite your close contacts along. This will give you a good opportunity to say farewell and share your plans with the people you have worked with.

Retirement will also free up time to make contact with old friends you maybe haven't spoken to in a long time because of work commitments or maybe because you have relocated for work. My wife and I moved from the city of Glasgow to the relatively small town of Dumfries 80 miles away for my work when I was in my early 30's and we had just got married and over time I lost contact with most of the friends I had so it is in my plans to make contact with some of them again rekindle those old friendships. Don't forget to include family members you may have lost contact with too. Use social media to find old friends and family you haven't seen for a long time.

It's also worth saying a few quick words on divorce here. According to nimblefins.co.uk the average overall divorce rate in England and Wales is 33.3%, based on all marriages between 1964 to 2019. However, the rate changes according to how many years a couple have been together. For example, of couples who married in 1967, only 31.9% had ended in divorce by 2017. In contrast, 43.6% of those marrying in 1987 had divorced by 2017. And 20.1% of couples married in 2007 had divorced within the first ten years. Divorce rates tended to increase until couples were married for 30 years and then declined after that. In 2019 the highest number of divorces peaked in people between the ages of 45 to 49 and then declined. However for all married couples over the age of 30, the over 60's group represent those with the lowest divorce rates. You'll be spending a lot more time with your partner so having patience and giving each other space and time to adjust to your retirement is an important consideration. Particularly if your partner is already retired, works from home or doesn't work. The human urge to feel useful and having meaningful things to do might lead you to dangerous encroachment into your spouse's territory on the home front. That's not to say you shouldn't be doing more on the domestic front. You probably should. Just don't move in on someone else's patch without their say so. Look at it as an amicable merger of responsibilities rather than a hostile takeover.

Dementia

The ONS reported that dementia and Alzheimer disease was the leading cause of death in 2018, accounting for 12.7% of all deaths registered in the UK. Research shows there are more than 850,000 people in the UK who have dementia. According to the NHS, 1 in 14 people over the age of 65 have dementia, and the condition affects 1 in 6 people over 80. The number of people with dementia is increasing because people are living longer. In addition, a better understanding of dementia and improved diagnosis is likely to have caused increased reporting of dementia on death certificates. It is estimated that by 2025, the number of people with dementia in the UK will be more than 1 million. According to a study by Dr Adrienne Tin from the University of Mississippi Medical Center, those who are active, eat well, lose weight, do not smoke, and keep their blood pressure, cholesterol and blood sugar under control are up to 43 per cent less likely to develop the condition. Whilst it's normal for your memory to be affected by stress, poor sleep, certain illnesses and medicines, if you are becoming increasingly forgetful, particularly if you're over the age of 65, it's a good idea to talk to a GP about the early signs of dementia. Although there is no cure for dementia at the moment, an early diagnosis means its progress can be slowed down in some cases, so you may be able to maintain your mental function for longer. An early diagnosis can help you get the right treatment and support as well as helping the people close to you, to prepare for the future.

Step 10 - Being Charitable with Your Time

'We make a living by what we get but we make a life by what we give' - Winston Churchill

I thought it was better to dedicate a (very short) Step to Volunteering on its own rather than including it in Step 6 about finding meaningful things to do because of the personal benefits I believe that volunteering and working for a charity give you. Especially, if like me, you haven't really done much of it before.

Like me you may have a few charities you have supported financially throughout your working life. Mine were the RSPCA and Poppy Scotland and my support was always in the form of cash donations. Some directly to the charities and some through my employers give as you earn schemes to maximise the tax benefits. I've also regularly donated books, toys and clothes to local charity shops. My biggest personal effort was to cycle from my employer's office in Glasgow to Cockenzie Power Station in East Lothian with two work colleagues when I was in my 40's. It was a 60 mile cycle but we got lost in Edinburgh (my fault) so it was 65 miles by the time we finished. We raised money for a local children's group and I remember a young woman who worked for the Charity meeting us at the finish to say thanks which was an unexpected welcome. What added to the fun was the fact that the wind was against us for the entire journey and cycling through rush hour traffic, not only as we left Glasgow but also as we arrived in Edinburgh. I was used to cycling in remote areas in the south of Scotland where you only need to worry about navigating past the odd tractor or wayward sheep!

Retirement brings the opportunity of donating something more valuable than cash though. Your time. Have a look at the websites of the charities close to your heart and see what opportunities there are for volunteering. You might want to use your personal or work related skills and knowledge or you might want to try something completely new.

Before I retired I had applied to 4 charities for a variety of different volunteering. It was just as rigorous as applying for a paid job in that there were initial written applications followed up by a telephone call or online interview, then usually a face to face interview followed up by personal reference and PVG checks. Be aware that charities operate just like employers in terms of the training courses you are required to do upfront. Something I was looking forward to leaving behind to be honest but they are a necessary hurdle to get over before you can start doing some of the good stuff.

Whatever it is you choose, giving up your time for a good cause will benefit your mental health and wellbeing, knowing that you are giving something back to society, to your local community or to a good cause close to your heart. Studies have shown charitable giving and helping others elicits a release of dopamine and endorphins - people who gave more to others in both time and resources also experienced greater satisfaction in life than people who did not. People who volunteered also scored better on key measurements in overall health, such as resilience during physical activity and blood pressure levels, than people who did not. Older adults who volunteered their time have also shown improved cognitive function, increased physical abilities and decreased rates of television watching than people who did not volunteer. So you're not only helping others by volunteering, you're helping your own health and wellbeing too!

Step 11 - Put Your Affairs in Order

'Make things as simple as possible but no simpler' - Albert Einstein

There are a number of things worth reviewing and considering to ensure that your legal and financial affairs are in order and that your spouse/partner/next of kin/children are up to date with your affairs should you become ill, incapacitated or die and are unable to deal with your affairs personally. I have ranked them in order of importance (although not necessarily in the order in which I dealt with them). Again I must say again I am not offering financial or legal advice here. I am giving you some things to think about. You should always seek professional independent financial and legal advice for your own situation and remember that the laws are different for the different parts of the UK. I've put links in the resources section to the relevant UK Government websites for the financial and legal matters that you can refer to for further information and updates.

Powers of Attorney POA - A lasting power of attorney (LPA) is a legal document that lets you (the 'donor') appoint one or more people (known as 'attorneys') to help you make decisions or to make decisions on your behalf. This gives you more control over what happens to you if you have an accident or an illness and cannot make your own decisions (if you 'lack mental capacity').

There are two types of Powers of Attorney and the laws are different in Scotland and the rest of the UK

Health and Welfare Lasting Power of Attorney

Use this LPA to give an attorney the power to make decisions about things like:

- your daily routine, for example washing, dressing, eating
- medical care
- moving into a care home
- life-sustaining treatment

An LPA can only be used when you're unable to make your own decisions.

Property and Financial Affairs Lasting Power of Attorney

Use this LPA to give an attorney the power to make decisions about money and property for you, for example:

- managing a bank or building society account
- paying bills
- collecting benefits or a pension
- selling your home

It can be used as soon as it's registered, with your permission.

Choosing An Attorney

You can choose one or more people to be your attorney. If you appoint more than one, you must decide whether they'll make decisions separately or together. You must appoint someone who has the mental capacity to make their own decisions. Your attorney does not need to live in the UK or be a British citizen.They could be:

- a relative
- a friend
- a professional, for example a solicitor
- your husband, wife or partner

When choosing an attorney, think about:

- how well they look after their own affairs, for example their finances
- how well you know them
- if you trust them to make decisions in your best interests
- how happy they will be to make decisions for you

You cannot choose someone who is subject to a Debt Relief Order or is bankrupt if you are making a lasting power of attorney (LPA) for property and financial affairs.

Wills

A will lets you decide what happens to your money, property and possessions after your death. If you make a will you can also make sure you do not pay more inheritance tax than you need to. You can write your will yourself, but it's probably best to seek legal advice particularly if your affairs are more complex. You need to get your will formally witnessed and signed to make it legally valid. If you want to update your will, you need to make an official alteration (called a 'codicil') or make a new will. If you die without a will, the law will decide who gets what. Keep your will safe. You can keep your will at your home or store it with your solicitor, your bank, a company that offers the storage of wills. You should also tell your executor (the person you've chosen to carry out your will), a close friend or relative where your will is.

Your will should lay out:

- who you want to benefit from your will, including charities
- who should look after any children under 18
- who is going to sort out your estate and carry out your wishes after your death (your executor)
- what happens if the people you want to benefit die before you

Dying without a Will

Understandably, no one likes to talk about death. Dying without a will is known as dying 'intestate', a word with Latin origins which essentially means 'without a testament'. It doesn't matter how close you are to certain relatives; if no will is made before you die, your assets and money will be allocated according to the same intestacy rules as anyone else. It is not up to your family to decide what happens. Spouses do not automatically inherit everything. If you die without writing a will, your property and money will be shared out according to a legal default, rather than your own expressed wishes.

Living Wills - Advance Decision - End of Life Care

An advance decision (sometimes known as an advance decision to refuse treatment, an ADRT, or a living will) is a decision you can make now to refuse a specific type of treatment at some time in the future. It lets your family, carers and health professionals know your wishes about refusing treatment if you're unable to make or communicate those decisions yourself. The treatments you're deciding to refuse must all be named in the advance decision. You may want to refuse a treatment in some situations, but not others. If this is the case, you need to be clear about all the circumstances in which you want to refuse this treatment. Deciding to refuse a treatment is not the same as asking someone to end your life or help you end your life. Euthenasia and assisted suicide are both illegal in the UK.

Care Home Costs

In the UK, on average, older people stay in a residential care home for 30 months. Paying for residential care in a care home is expensive and again the rules are different in the different parts of the UK. How much you will pay for your care depends on where you live, what type of care you need, your savings, assets and the care home provider itself. Being aware of the cost of care home fees will help you make important decisions about your own or a loved one's care. In May 2022 the average monthly cost of living in a residential care home was £2,816, whilst the average nursing home cost is £3,552 across the UK. So the average total cost of staying in a care home for 30 months would be £84,480 and a nursing home would be £106,560. Compare this to say the average cost for a three year university degree of £57,000 or with the average first-time buyer's deposit currently estimated at £33,000 and you can see it's a significant outgoing in comparison to the other one off big expenses you will have in your lifetime.

There is some help available to meet the cost of care, but the care system can be complicated and difficult to navigate. You may be eligible for financial help from your local council or, in some circumstances, from the NHS. If you are eligible for funding support, your local council could pay some or most of the fees. The council will carry out a care needs assessment. If this concludes you need care in a care home, they will carry out a means test to work out whether you qualify for help with the cost. This will look at your income and capital. The council must ensure that the overall cost figure it calculates, called the 'personal budget', is high enough to meet the cost of at least one suitable care home. You will be expected to pay towards the cost from your income included in the financial assessment, however you must be left a Personal Expenses Allowance.

Some people take actions such as equity release and gifting assets to relatives so that they appear to have less money in assets than they do in reality, with the aim of reducing the amount they have to pay for care. Whilst the deprivation of assets is not an uncommon practice, it is not recommended. Before being means tested, most local authorities will look to see if such actions have taken place.

www.carehome.co.uk is a good source of information on care homes.

Inheritance Tax Planning

In the UK, significant changes to Inheritance Tax (IHT) rules were announced in the winter budget of 2024, affecting Business Property Relief (BPR) and Agricultural Property Relief (APR), as well as the taxation of pension funds and death benefits.

Business Property Relief (BPR) and Agricultural Property Relief (APR): Effective from 6 April 2026, the government will cap the 100% relief available under BPR and APR to the first £1 million of qualifying assets. Assets exceeding this threshold will receive a reduced relief rate of 50%, resulting in an effective IHT rate of 20% on the excess value. Notably, unlisted shares, including those listed on the Alternative Investment Market (AIM), will only qualify for the 50% relief, regardless of their value.

Taxation of Pension Funds and Death Benefits: Starting from 6 April 2027, most unused pension funds and death benefits payable from a pension will be included within an individual's estate for IHT purposes. Pension scheme administrators will be responsible for reporting and paying any IHT due. This change aims to prevent pensions from being used primarily as vehicles for accumulating capital sums intended for inheritance.

Extension of Nil-Rate Bands: The freeze on the IHT nil-rate band (£325,000) and the residence nil-rate band (£175,000) has been extended until 5 April 2030. This means that qualifying estates can continue to pass on up to £500,000 tax-free, and up to £1 million for qualifying estates of a surviving spouse or civil partner.

Transition from Domicile-Based to Residency-Based Taxation: From 6 April 2025, the UK will shift from a domicile-based to a residency-based system for determining IHT liability. Individuals who have been UK residents for at least 10 years will be subject to IHT on their worldwide assets. Additionally, those who become non-UK residents will remain within the scope of IHT for a further 10 years, referred to as the '10-year tail.'

These reforms are part of the government's efforts to make the IHT system fairer and more targeted, particularly affecting larger estates and certain investments. Individuals and trustees are advised to review their estate planning strategies in light of these changes.

Minimizing inheritance tax (IHT) in the UK requires careful planning and adherence to legal rules. Here are some strategies people use to reduce their inheritance tax liability:

1. Understand the Thresholds

- The **nil-rate band (NRB)** is £325,000, meaning estates below this value are not taxed.
- The **residence nil-rate band (RNRB)** provides an additional allowance (up to £175,000 in 2023/24) if a primary residence is left to direct descendants.

2. Gifting Assets

- **Annual Exemption:** You can gift up to £3,000 each tax year free of IHT. If unused, it can be carried forward one year.

- **Small Gift Allowance:** You can give up to £250 per person annually, free of IHT.
- **Wedding Gifts:** You can give tax-free gifts for weddings, e.g., £5,000 to a child, £2,500 to a grandchild, and £1,000 to others.
- **Potentially Exempt Transfers (PETs):** Gifts made more than seven years before death are generally exempt. A taper relief applies if death occurs between three and seven years.

3. Use Trusts

- Setting up **trusts** allows you to transfer assets out of your estate while maintaining control under specific conditions. Trusts can be complex and require professional advice.

4. Leave Money to Charity

- Bequests to registered charities are IHT-free. If you leave at least 10% of your estate to charity, the IHT rate on the remainder may reduce from 40% to 36%.

5. Business and Agricultural Relief

- Business property and certain agricultural property may qualify for **Business Relief** or **Agricultural Relief**, reducing their value for IHT purposes by up to 100%.

6. Invest in Exempt Assets

- Investments in **Enterprise Investment Schemes (EIS)** and certain other qualifying assets may become

IHT-free after two years if they are held at the time of death.

7. Life Insurance Policies

- Take out a life insurance policy to cover IHT liability and place it in a trust so the payout does not form part of the estate.

8. Joint Ownership of Assets

- Ensure property ownership is structured efficiently, such as **tenants in common**, so part of the property can be passed on using exemptions.

10. Regular Lifetime Gifts from Income

- Gifts made from surplus income (not capital) can be IHT-free if they are regular and do not reduce your standard of living.

11. Update Wills and Use Professional Advice

- A well-structured **will** ensures assets are distributed efficiently.
- Seek advice from an estate planning professional or solicitor for tailored strategies.

Insurance Policies

Your employer might have provided you with life or health insurance when you worked with them. You will lose this protection in retirement so review all of your life, critical illness and health insurance policies to see if they are still appropriate and meet your needs. If you have paid off all of your debts, your children have flown the nest and you have sufficient assets and pension funds etc. then perhaps you don't need as much insurance cover as you did when you were working. You might want to consider continuing with your existing policies until they expire and then leave it at that.

Step 12 - Write Your Own Bucket List

'Twenty years from now you will be more disappointed by the things you didn't do than by the ones you did. So throw off the bowlines, sail away from the safe harbour. Catch the trade winds in your sails. Explore. Dream. Discover' - Mark Twain. No book on retirement would be complete without talking about bucket lists. For me, this has been one of the best parts of retirement and also for researching the book. Your bucket list items could be the things that you've never had the time, the finances or the freedom to pursue when you were working. Your aspirational goals. There are plenty of bucket lists online where you can get ideas from and I have provided a few links to suggested websites to have a look at below. I have summarised and briefly discussed the most common and popular things on the various bucket lists that I have researched. It might be useful to have your own bucket list printed out and pinned to a wall or your fridge so you don't forget about it and where you can refer to it for ideas and start making arrangements and planning things in your diary at the same time.

Bucket Lists

- 101 Fun Things to Do in Retirement - Stella Rheingold
- https://www.ageukmobility.co.uk/mobility-news/article/retirement-bucket-list
- https://www.maturetimes.co.uk/ultimate-retirement-bucket-list/

Flying, Cruising and Driving

Travelling is a high priority on many retirees bucket list and includes everything from going on cruises, train journeys, bus tours, visiting countries and cities you have never been to before, going on safari, driving Route 66, the SouthWest660 or the NorthCoast500 in the in a motorhome or motorbikes even.

- https://www.forbes.com/sites/ericrosen/2019/11/12/the-2020-list-of-the-worlds-best-cruises-is-out-now/
- https://www.lonelyplanet.com/articles/worlds-most-amazing-train-journeys
- https://www.timeout.com/things-to-do/best-cities-in-the-world
- https://www.northcoast500.com/
- https://southwest660.com/route
- https://www.wandering-bird.com/motorhome-holidays-uk/

Walking, Hiking and Cycling

Walking, hiking and cycling tours are another common favourite on retirement bucket lists. You could do these as days out or as part of a tour with overnight stays in local B&B's or even with your rucksack and tent.

- https://theoutdoorguide.co.uk/britains-favourite-walks/
- https://www.walkhighlands.co.uk/
- https://westhighlandway.com/
- https://www.visitscotland.com/see-do/active/walking/munro-bagging/
- https://www.nationaltrust.org.uk/features/hill-and-mountain-walks
- https://europeancyclingtours.com/

Living Abroad

Another favourite on the bucket list of many retirees is to move abroad or at least experience some time living abroad. Preferably somewhere warmer than the UK. This could involve you selling up and moving abroad permanently or keeping your home and renting a property abroad for a few months each year. If you are considering buying an overseas property it's important you do all of your research and consider everything including healthcare, visas, driving rules and licence requirements, tax rules, utilities, tax, bank accounts, currency, exchange rates, pets and of course learning the language.

- https://expatra.com/articles/living-abroad/best-countries-to-retire/
- https://britishexpatguide.co.uk/10-best-places-to-retire-overseas/
- https://www.expertsforexpats.com/relocation/moving-abroad-checklist/

Movies, Documentaries, Books, Audio Books, Podcasts and Music

And then of course for those quiet days or when the weather isn't great for being outside there are all the great movies, books and music albums you haven't had the time to watch, read or listen to in a while.

- https://www.timeout.com/film/best-movies-of-all-time
- https://www.thetimes.co.uk/article/best-documentaries-you-have-to-see-dnkp5zgmw
- https://www.goodreads.com/list/show/2681.Time_Magazine_s_All_Time_100_Novels

- https://www.alltopeverything.com/top-10-most-popular-podcasts/
- https://www.rollingstone.com/music/music-lists/best-albums-of-all-time-1062063/

Live Sporting Events

Maybe you've always wanted to see a live sporting or cultural event. Wimbledon, the Grand National, the Grand Prix, Le Mans, the Football World Cup, the Champions League, the Olympics, the Six Nations Rugby, the Tour de France, the Giro D'Italia, the Masters Snooker, the Super Bowl, the Masters Golf Tournament, the Ryder Cup, the World Darts Championship, the options are unlimited.

https://www.topendsports.com/world/lists/must-see-events/top100.htm

Live Cultural Events

Theatre, Comedy, Dance, Opera, Concerts and Music Festivals

- https://www.timeout.com/newyork/theater/best-plays-of-all-time
- https://www.timeout.com/music/the-50-best-music-festivals-in-the-world
- https://www.edfringe.com/
- https://www.roh.org.uk/

Personal Challenges

How about setting yourself some personal challenges that you never had the time to pursue when you were working? Study for a degree, learn to speak a new language, write a book, learn to play an instrument, run a marathon, cycle a stage of the Tour De France or even a local Sportive, enter a triathlon race, climb a mountain or some of Scotland's Munros or do a long distance walk. You could combine your personal challenge with a charity fundraiser too.

Getting a Dog (or a Cat)

If you've never owned a dog (or a cat) then retirement is probably one of the best times to do it. You will have the time to give the animal the love, care and attention it needs and in return it will provide you with companionship, happiness, exercise, responsibility and love.

- https://www.dogstrust.org.uk/help-advice/buyer-advice/
- https://www.rspca.org.uk/adviceandwelfare/pets/dogs/puppy
- https://www.cats.org.uk/adopt-a-cat

12 Step Summary

I have recapped some of the key points from my 12 step retirement plan below as a reminder and to help you manage your own plans.

Step 1 - Why Should You Retire

Write down the reasons why you want to retire, your retirement alternatives, what you won't miss and what you will miss about work. Think about what you want to do to replace the things you will miss about work. Weigh these factors up, review them with your family and decide if your reasons are strong enough for retiring. If your only reasons for retiring are because you can, financially speaking, and you don't like your job, then you might find you don’t like retirement much either unless you've made a robust plan and you have meaningful things to fill your time. Many people spend more time planning their annual holiday than they do their own retirement.

Step 2 - How Much Is Enough

Work out your net financial worth including savings, assets, pensions and liabilities and decide if these are sufficient enough to meet your financial Needs, Wants and Aspirations in retirement. Everyone's answer to how much is enough will be different of course and only you can decide how much is enough for you. If you are willing to make some lifestyle sacrifices and cut backs then you can probably retire sooner.

Step 3 - Pension Options

Review your pensions in conjunction with your other assets and consider the best options for crystallising them in a manner that is both tax efficient and ensures they will last you throughout your retirement. If you have a defined contribution or personal pension then you could apply the 4% rule as a rough guide to calculate what your annual pension could be and don't forget about the state pension. Speak to an independent financial adviser.

Step 4 - When Should You Retire

Focus on the things within your own sphere of influence. Don't worry about things you can't control. You don't have control over natural disasters, wars, pandemics, inflation, interest rates, the stock market or your genetic disposition. There are so many things you do not have control over, if you are waiting for all of the stars to align in your favour it will be your funeral, not your retirement, you're planning for. Consider your life expectancy based on personal health, lifestyle and family history. Focus on the things you have control over such as the lifestyle you want to lead, how much money you want to spend, where you want to live, how much you want to help your children and grandchildren financially, where your assets are invested and how healthy a life you want to lead.

Step 5 - Slowing Things Down

Don't retire on Friday and wake up on Monday with nothing to do. Consider the first stage of retirement as a slowing down phase by working part time or reducing your working week from 5 to 4 to 3 days if you can. Give at least 1 year's retirement notice. Expand your retirement activities, hobbies and interests at the same time. But make sure you're not doing 5 days work in a 3 day week though! Consciously step down a gear or 2. If you find that you're not really enjoying the additional days off or that you are happy just working part time then there might still be an option to stay at work in this capacity.

Step 6 - Pursue Meaningful Things

It is in responsibility that most people find the meaning that sustains them through life. Take on new responsibilities, challenging activities and replace work goals with personal ones. Write down your short, medium and long term goals and review them regularly. These could be personal, health, family, relationship, social, financial, educational, societal and charitable goals. Write your own biography and then someone else's. story. Become a Minimalist and declutter your life of unnecessary possessions. Find meaning and a sense of identity from who you are rather than from what you own.

Step 7 - Creating a New Routine

Create a new routine for your new life. Having a routine will help you cope with the changes that you will experience in retirement. It will help you create healthy habits, avoid bad ones and reduce stress levels. When you are organised and have a set routine, you know what to expect. This takes the anxiety out of thinking about what is coming next. Routines can liberate your mental health and bring psychological benefits including alleviating symptoms of mental disorders and insomnia. Use a wall calendar or a phone app to plan and keep track of appointments, holidays, activities and give you things to look forward to. It doesn't have to be rigid and don't be a slave to it or allow it to dampen spontaneity or get in the way of the opportunities that come your way.

Step 8 - Looking After Your Physical Health

The benefits of physical exercise at any age are well documented. Current guidelines from health professionals say that engaging in around 150 minutes of moderate intensity activity or 75 minutes of vigorous intensity activity per week decreases the risk of mortality by 27%. Physical activity reduces many major mortality risk factors including arterial hypertension, type 2 diabetes, dyslipidemia, coronary heart disease, stroke, and cancer. Exercise also improves mental health and improves sleep quality by reducing anxiety, depression, improving cognitive function and has also been found to alleviate symptoms such as low self-esteem and social withdrawal. Focus on your functional fitness - doing movements that mimic everyday actions, incorporating multiple muscle groups at the same time. This builds strength, stability and mobility across the body, making us more efficient human beings not only inside the gym but outside as well.

Step 9 - Looking After Your Mental Health

There will be emotional ups and downs as you transition from your life in work to your new life in retirement. Feelings of apprehension, anxiety and sometimes depression are not unusual in retirement. The emotional transition of retiring is not dissimilar to the other significant events we experience in life such as marriage, divorce, redundancy, serious illness, injury or even the death of a loved one. Look at maintaining existing relationships as well as making new ones. Look at techniques for practising mindfulness, creating habits for getting a good night's sleep and focusing on building resilience. Think about your new sense of identity and what you are going to say when people ask you what you do when you no longer have a job to talk about. Update your social media profiles. Be mindful of the dangers of loneliness and do not be ashamed, afraid or embarrassed to seek help or emotional support.

Step 10 - Being Charitable with Your Time

Giving up your time for a good cause will benefit your mental health and wellbeing. Studies have shown that charitable giving and helping others elicits a release of dopamine and endorphins. People who give or do more for others experience greater satisfaction in life than people who do not. People who volunteer also score better on key measurements in overall health, such as resilience during physical activity and blood pressure levels, than people who do not. Older adults who volunteer their time show improved cognitive function, increased physical abilities and decreased rates of television watching than people who do not volunteer.

Step 11 - Putting Things in Order

Review your will and power of attorney documents with a good solicitor. Make sure your family is aware of all of your affairs, investments, assets, insurance policies and how you want things dealt with in the event of your death or incapacity. Consider how you might pay for care home fees and review your inheritance tax plans.

Step 12 - Writing Your Own Bucket List

Research and draw up a personal bucket list. Think about things you would like to do that you never had the time, freedom or finances to do when you were working. Pin it on the wall somewhere where you can see it and tick off as you complete them and add new ones to replace them.

Epilogue

'Non - Je Ne Regrette Rien' - Edith Piaf

An essay in the Times from April 2022 by Emma Duncan called - 'why getting older can mean having the time of your life', discussed the popular assumption that the young have all the fun but the reality is that, once you've survived the stressful middle years, the next three decades are the ones likely to bring you the most happiness. Dante's passage through Hell and Purgatory to Heaven is most obviously a religious experience but you can also read it as a journey from the hardest part of life to the best. Andrew Oswald, a professor of economics at the University of Warwick researched data on how people felt about their lives, and found that it confirmed Dante's perception that middle age was a dark place. Most people, when asked what period of life they were most happiest in, chose youth. However the life-satisfaction scores of Britons start climbing in their 40's and continue to rise for three decades and people are most satisfied with life in their 70s. Older people are also much less prone to depression or anxiety than the young and the middle-aged and also less likely to be prescribed antidepressants.

As I was writing the first edition of the book I was also planning for and also going through my own retirement experience so it had been a work in progress over 12 months. At the point of writing the second edition I am into my third year of retirement and have come through the emotional ups and downs and made the adjustments from full time employment and feel more settled now.

I was thinking of what to write in the Epilogue during 2 very wet days in July of my initial months of retirement and I realised that, had I still been working, I would have been in a very different frame of mind on those days. People who know me from work will understand why I would have wanted to write this passage. The life of an Hydro-Electric Scheme Operations Manager often involves the neurotic examination of weather forecasts for potential flooding events and then modelling what this might look like for the scheme's dams, reservoirs and stakeholders. This would normally include having numerous updates and calls with the emergency services, the local authority emergency teams, the environment agency and local stakeholders who might be affected by flooding. This was a big part of my job and it did cause me a fair degree of stress and a few sleepless nights (flooding always seemed to happen during the night) so I think it's worth mentioning here to reflect on one of the things I definitely don't miss about my job! To be honest I think it was the first time I'd really thought about my work since retiring and I did send a few messages to my old colleagues wishing them the best of luck with these 2 wet days in July.

But it still doesn't really feel like 'proper' retirement to me yet, although it's still early days. My wife still has another 2 years until she can retire (if she does that is), my son has another 2 years at High School and my daughter is just about to finish University so it will probably be another 6 years or so before we both have the kind of freedom to do some of our bucket list items. But until that time comes and for the moment, I have left all of my work related worries, stress and anxieties behind me. I am sleeping better, eating better, exercising more, feeling fitter, happier, healthier, more relaxed and generally keeping busy, enjoying myself and looking forward to what the future holds. Don't get me wrong there are still times when I think of what I have left behind. I do occasionally miss the relationships, responsibility, routine and the daily challenges that my full time job provided. It sometimes still feels like there is a little bit of a void to fill, however I am doing this gradually with my volunteering and my fitness activities as well as just enjoying the freedom to do whatever I want for now really. And who knows what the future will bring. I wouldn't rule out doing some form of paid work again. It would probably have to be something on a part time basis though. But for the moment I've got enough on my hands to keep me busy.

Hopefully my book has been useful for you and will help you along the road to planning your own retirement. Just remember we are all luckier now that we have ever been from a retirement perspective. We are all living longer, happier, healthier and wealthier retirements than our parents and grandparents ever did. If there's one thing you take away from this book it's that you should plan for your retirement. Don't just walk into it blindly. Give serious thought to the impact that retirement will have on you and your family, not just financially but also from a health and wellbeing perspective too. You've worked for it so best of luck and I hope you make it to your own retirement heaven one day soon!

Acknowledgements

Thanks to my family, friends and work colleagues for their encouragement and feedback in writing the book.

Resources

Step 1 - Why Should You Retire

- https://www.thetimes.co.uk/article/over-50s-are-retiring-in-droves-but-will-they-be-forced-back-into-work-ml8fm9mbq

Step 2 - How Much is Enough

- The Psychology of Money: Timeless lessons on wealth, greed, and happiness - Morgan Housel
- https://www.nimblefins.co.uk/savings-accounts/average-household-savings-uk
- https://www.retirementlivingstandards.org.uk/
- https://www.gov.uk/plan-retirement-income/get-financial-advice
- https://youtube.com/c/MeaningfulMoneyUK

Step 3 - Pension Options

- https://www.gov.uk/check-state-pension
- https://www.which.co.uk/money/pensions-and-retirement/options-for-cashing-in-your-pensions/income-drawdown/income-drawdown-calculator-making-your-money-last-awvp49g8uq6l
- https://www.moneyhelper.org.uk/en/pensions-and-retirement/pensions-basics/use-our-pension-calculator
- https://www.pensionsarchive.org.uk/76/
- https://currentmarketvaluation.com/models/buffett-indicator.php
- https://helpandadvice.co.uk/final-salary-pension-transfer/

Step 3 - When Should You Retire

- https://www.ons.gov.uk/peoplepopulationandcommunity/healthandsocialcare/healthandlifeexpectancies/articles/lifeexpectancycalculator/2019-06-07

Step 5 - Slowing things Down

https://retirebydegrees.com/

Step 6 - Pursue Meaningful Things

- 12 Rules for Life - An Antidote to Chaos - Jordan Peterson
- https://www.selfauthoring.com
- https://substack.com/
- https://www.u3a.org.uk/
- https://www.wondrium.com/
- https://www.theminimalists.com/

Step 7 - Create a New Routine

- 4000 Weeks - Time and How to Use it - Oliver Burkeman
- https://www.realsimple.com/work-life/life-strategies/benefits-of-routines
- https://www.skilledatlife.com/18-reasons-why-a-daily-routine-is-so-important/

Step 8 - Looking After Your Physical Health

- https://www.youtube.com/watch?v=A2wp8Ipxn9s
- https://www.youtube.com/watch?v=7aHK2sgjBCM
- https://www.verywellfit.com/the-best-exercises-for-core-strength-3120054
- https://www.thetimes.co.uk/article/importance-of-balance-8082t0kv8
- https://podcasts.apple.com/gb/podcast/feel-better-live-more-with-dr-rangan-chatterjee/id1333552422
- https://bestlifeonline.com/building-muscle-after-50/

- https://www.nhs.uk/live-well/healthy-weight/bmi-calculator/
- https://www.finder.com/uk/health-insurance-statistics
- https://www.bluecrestwellness.com/

Step 9 - Looking After Your Mental Health

- Why We Sleep - Mathew Walker
- https://grief.com/the-five-stages-of-grief/
- https://youtube.com/watch?v=DMHMOQ_054U&feature=share
- https://www.wakingup.com/
- https://www.mind.org.uk/
- https://wavelength.org.uk/
- https://www.sleep.org/
- https://www.redcross.org.uk/get-help/get-help-with-loneliness/wellbeing-support/resilience-building-activities
- https://www.nimblefins.co.uk/divorce-statistics-uk
- https://www.nhs.uk/conditions/dementia/about/

Step 10 - Being Charitable with Your Time

- https://www.charitychoice.co.uk/charities
- https://www.ageuk.org.uk/

Step 11 - Putting Things in Order

- https://www.gov.uk/power-of-attorney
- https://www.gov.uk/make-will
- https://www.gov.uk/inheritance-tax
- https://www.carehome.co.uk/advice/fees
- https://helpandadvice.co.uk/

Epilogue

https://www.thetimes.co.uk/article/why-getting-older-can-mean-having-the-time-of-your-life-dpgm0drrs

Other Resources

Joe Kuhn
https://www.youtube.com/channel/UCY0hd1Iff79JnPNkPHmOXAg

Roger Whitney
https://retirementpodcastnetwork.com/podcasts/retirement-answer-man/

Fritz Gilbert
https://www.theretirementmanifesto.com/

Printed in Dunstable, United Kingdom

67092047R00070